Supplement to 'Basic Research in Cardiology', Vol. 79 (1984)

The symposium was held under the auspices of the **Arbeitsgruppe positiv inotrope Pharmaka** der Deutschen Gesellschaft für Herz- und Kreislaufforschung and the **Working group Drug Therapy in Cardiology** of the European Society of Cardiology.

Supplement to
"Basic Research in Cardiology", Vol. 79 (1984)
Editors: R. Jacob (Tübingen) and W. Schaper (Bad Nauheim)

Cardiac Glycoside Receptors and Positive Inotropy

Evidence for more than one receptor?

Symposium, Munich, October 26–29, 1983

Editor: E. Erdmann (Munich)

With Contributions by L. Brown, W. H. Barry, D. Charlemagne, E. Erdmann, A. A. L. Fox, U. Fricke, W. H. van Gilst, T. Godfraind, K. Greeff, M. Heller, K.-O. Haustein, G. Isenberg, R. Jacob, T. Kazazoglou, D. Kim, K. Kochsiek, J. M. Koomen, W. Krawietz, M. Lazdunski, L. G. Lelievre, H. Lüllmann, P. Mansier, E. Noack, D. Noble, D. Palm, Th. Peters, H.-H. Prillwitz, J. F. Renaud, B. Rossi, J. A. M. Schevers, Th. W. Smith, W. Schmitz, H. Scholz, B. Swynghedauw, B. Wagenknecht, M. F. Wendt-Gallitelli, A. Wellstein, K. Werdan, J. Wilting, A. Ziegler, B. Zwißler

Steinkopff Verlag · Darmstadt

ISSN 0175-9418
ISBN-13:978-3-642-72378-0 e-ISBN-13:978-3-642-72376-6
DOI: 10.1007/978-3-642-72376-6

Softcover reprint of the hardcover 1st edition 1984

Contents

Cardiac glycoside receptors and positive inotropy Evidence for more than one receptor?

E. Erdmann (München)

Editorial

Biochemists, pharmacologists and electrophysiologists have produced quite controversial experimental results during the last 30 years for the hypothetical mode of action of cardiac glycosides in the heart. This is rather astonishing since it began very straight forward: Schatzmann (14) discovered that cardiac glycosides specifically inhibit the active Na^+/K^+-transport system of the erythrocyte; Skou (15) could demonstrate that the $(Na^+ + K^+)$-ATPase is the enzymatic basis for the active transport of Na^+ and K^+ across cell membranes and this enzyme is specifically inhibited by cardiac glycosides. Therefore, Repke (12) called this enzyme the digitalis receptor and after a great many experiments, he formulated a theory explaining the mode of action of cardiac glycosides by 1. an inhibition of the $(Na^+ + K^+)$-ATPase, which 2. would lead to intracellular losses of K^+ and accumulation of Na^+, the latter 3. would cause an increase of intracellular Ca^{++}, which in turn would 4. stimulate the contractile proteins to a larger extent than before addition of the drugs. This hypothesis seemed to explain the increase in force of contraction rather well and also the clinically important arrhythmias, which were considered to be related to an almost complete inhibition of the $(Na^+ + K^+)$-ATPase. Numerous workers indeed did find raised intracellular Na^+ in digitalis-intoxicated cardiac preparations – not, however, in low but nevertheless positive inotropic concentrations of glycosides.

When Matsui and Schwartz (10) measured specific ^3H-digoxin binding to $(Na^+ + K^+)$-ATPase preparations from calf heart, this finding seemed to support the above mentioned hypothesis of Repke, because further experiments showed that the $(Na^+ + K^+)$-ATPase contains an α-subunit of about 96,000 daltons, that specifically binds cardiac glycosides according to the law of mass action (1). Reuter (13) then discovered a membrane bound Na^+-Ca^{++}-counter-transport system in the heart, that would fit nicely into this putative mode of action of digitalis by coupling the raised intracellular Ca^{++} to the augmented Na^+_i.

Thus, the mechanism of action of cardiac glycosides seemed to be elucidated. However, there were several pieces of evidence that did not fit into this hypothesis: electrophysiological experiments were interpreted as showing a stimulation of the Na^+/K^+-pump by low concentrations of cardiac glycosides (11). This interpretation was supported by biochemical work mainly by Godfraind and coworkers (2, 3). Others could not find, under those conditions, either a raised intracellular Na^+ or a decreased K^+ (8, 9).

If one interviewed scientists working in this field, they most likely would be split into 50 % agreeing with Repke's hypothesis, which had later been updated by Langer (4, 5), and 50 % questioning it, although some recent experiments with intracellular electrodes (6, 7) demonstrated clearly that cardiac glycosides in a concentration dependent way increase intracellular Na^+-activity in sheep and dog purkinje fibers.

Recently, several laboratories published experimental evidence for the existence of several types of cardiac glycoside receptors in the heart. In brain tissue, two different molecular forms of $(Na^+ + K^+)$-ATPase with different affinities for strophanthidin had been separated in 1979 by Sweadner (16). Thus, it is tempting to speculate on the significance of different cardiac glycoside receptors with functionally different roles in the complex ion transport mechanism of the heart. Some of the experimental results (stimulation or inhibition of the sodium pump etc.), at first sight contradictory, might be explained by the existence of several types of (Na^+ + K^+)-ATPases. Furthermore, there is ample evidence of species differences as rat and guinea pig are relatively digitalis insensitive whereas cat, calf, dog, sheep and human are digitalis sensitive. In order to discuss these problems freely and to critically review the evidence for or against the existence of functionally different types of cardiac glycoside receptors in the heart, we asked some of the most eminent scientists in this field to share their results in a symposium "Cardiac Glycoside Receptors and Positive Inotropy – evidence for more than one receptor?" (Munich, October 26–29, 1983).

The following papers are the manuscripts of this international meeting, which was made possible by the support of Boehringer Mannheim. I would like to express my gratitude for the generous help especially to Dr. med. Horst Wenzel from Boehringer, who realized that different types of digitalis receptors raise the possibility of more specific drugs for the treatment of cardiac failure.

This symposium, I think, established beyond doubt the existence of nonuniformity of digitalis receptors in the heart.

References

1. Erdmann E (1981) Influence of cardiac glycosides on their receptor. In: Greeff K (ed) Handb Exp Pharmacol, Vol 56/I (Springer Verlag Berlin Heidelberg), p 337–380
2. Godfraind T, Ghysel-Burton J (1980) Independence of the positive inotropic effect of ouabain from the inhibition of the heart Na^+/K^+ Pump. Proc Natl Acad Sci USA 77:3067–3069
3. Ghysel-Burton J, Godfraind T (1979) Stimulation and inhibition of the sodium pump by cardioactive steroids in relation to their binding sites and their inotropic effect on guinea-pig isolated atria. Br J Pharmacol 66:175–184
4. Langer GA (1977) Relationship between myocardial contractility and the effects of digitalis on ionic exchange. Fed Proc 36:2231–2234
5. Langer GA (1981) Mechanism of action of the cardiac glycosides on the heart. Biochem Pharmacol 30:3261–3264
6. Lee ChO, Kang DH, Sokol JH, Lee KS (1980) Relation between intracellular Na ion activity and tension of sheep cardiac purkinje fibers exposed to dihydro-ouabain. Biophys J 29:315–330
7. Lee ChO, Dagostino M (1982) Effect of strophanthin on intracellular Na ion activity and twitch tension of constantly driven canine cardiac purkinje fibers. Biophys J 40:185–198
8. Lee KS, Klaus W (1971) The subcellular basis for the mechanism of inotropic action of cardiac glycosides. Pharmacol Rev 23:193–261
9. Lüllmann H, Peters T (1979) Action of cardiac glycosides. Prog Pharmacol 2:5–57
10. Matsui H, Schwartz A (1968) Mechanism of cardiac glycoside inhibition of the (Na^+ + K^+)-dependent ATPase from cardiac tissue. Biochim Biophys Acta 151:655–663
11. Noble D (1980) Mechanism of action of therapeutic levels of cardiac glycoside. Cardiovasc. Res 14:495–514
12. Repke K, Est M, Portius HJ (1965) Über die Ursache der Speciesunterschiede in der Digitalisempfindlichkeit. Biochem Pharmacol 14:1785–1802
13. Reuter H (1974) Exchange of calcium ions in the mammalian myocardium. Mechanisms and physiological significance. Circ Res 34:599–605
14. Schatzmann HJ (1953) Herzglykoside als Hemmstoffe für den aktiven Kalium- und Natriumtransport durch die Erythrocytenmembran. Helv Physiol Acta 11:346–354
15. Skou JC (1957) The influence of some cations on an adenosine triphosphatase from peripheral nerves. Biochim Biophys Acta 23:349–401
16. Sweadner KJ (1979) Two molecular forms of (Na^+ + K^+)-stimulated ATPase in brain. J Biol Chem 254:6060–6070

Author's address:

Priv. Doz. Dr. med. E. Erdmann, Medizinische Klinik I der Universität München, Klinikum Großhadern, Marchioninistr. 15, 8000 München 70

Theory of ligand – receptor interactions – Evidence for more than one site*/**

A. Wellstein and D. Palm

Zentrum der Pharmakologie, Klinikum der J. W. Goethe-Universität Frankfurt/M, Frankfurt/M. (FRG)

Summary

Receptor binding studies usually show heterogenic characteristics of the binding isotherm. Scatchard transformation for graphical linearization of the data presentation affects the data inhomogeneously with respect to the experimental error. Thus a non-linear fitting procedure should be preferred for data analysis. Furthermore this approach allows for reliable weighting of the measurements according to the experimental error.

Key words: receptor binding, curve fitting, non-linear regression, ^{3}H-ouabain binding, multiple binding sites.

Introduction

Receptor binding studies with tritiated or iodinated radioligands of high affinity to their receptors have provided an ever increasing body of knowledge about ligand receptor interactions in different tissues, different species and at different receptors and receptor subtypes. Some problems arise, when the interaction cannot be described by one single bimolecular reaction on the basis of the law of mass action but rather multiple binding sites or receptor sites or cooperativity among the binding entities. In the following some basic problems of interpretation of such data shall be considered with special respect to multiple binding sites.

Methods

Two fundamental approaches to the investigation of ligand receptor interaction via receptor binding are possible (8):

(1) Equilibrium binding studies either incubating increasing concentrations of radioligand with the membrane suspension (saturation binding isotherm) or a fixed concentration of radioligand with increasing concentrations of non-labeled ligand (competition binding)

(2) Kinetic approach either incubating membrane suspensions with radioligand for different time intervals until steady state is achieved (association kinetics) or diluting suspensions after equilibration infinitely, alternatively adding excess of non-labeled ligand after equilibrium to measure dissociation of bound radioligand at different time intervals (dissociation kinetics).

The data of ^{3}H-ouabain binding were kindly provided by Dr. Erdmann and his coworkers (2). Binding of ^{3}H-N-methylscopolamine (NEN, Dreieich, 40–60 Ci/mmol) to rat parotid gland membranes was measured in 300 µl of TRIS-buffer (50 mmol/l, pH 7.4 at 25° C) containing 150–250 µg of membrane protein per vial incubated at 25° C for 60 minutes. Bound and free radioligand were separated by filtration through glass fiber filters (Millipore, Neu-Isenburg, AP 15) which were washed with 20 ml of buffer.

---

*Supported by a grant from the Deutsche Forschungsgemeinschaft. We wish to thank the Dr. Robert Pfleger Stiftung for support of our investigations.

**Dedicated to Prof. Lüllmann, Kiel on occasion of his 60th birthday.

Analysis of data was performed by a non-linear least square fitting procedure of the binding function to the measurements using the following equation according to (3):

$$(1)\ B = \sum_{i=1}^{n} \frac{B_{max,i,m} \times {}^3H}{{}^3H + K_{D^3H,i,m} \times (1 + \sum_{m=1}^{k} \frac{comp}{K_{Dcomp,m}})} + nsb \times {}^3H$$

where i and m represent the number of binding isotherms of the radioligand and non labeled competing ligand (comp). B_{max} and K_D are the capacity and half-maximal saturating ligand concentration resp. nsb is the slope of non-specific binding. ^3H and comp are concentrations of radioligand and competing ligand resp.

In the computations each data pair was given the mean variance of the replicative measurements of bound as a weight. If less than 3 replications were performed each data pair was given the weight of 1. The calculations were performed on a Hewlett-Packard 9826 desktop calculator using a HP-language program developed by D. Brockmeier and H. M. v. Hattingberg (c. f. 7).

Results and Discussion

The simplest case of interaction between a ligand (L) and receptor (R) can be described by the equation:

$$(2)\quad L + R \underset{k_{-1}}{\overset{k_{+1}}{\rightleftharpoons}} LR$$

At equilibrium one may write according to the law of mass action:

$$(3)\quad \frac{k_{-1}}{k_{+1}} = K_D = \frac{L \times R}{LR}$$

LR is measured in binding studies as "bound" (B), and R (the free receptor concentration) is equal to the total receptor concentration (B_{max}) minus B. Equation (3) can thus be rewritten as (4) $B = B_{max} \times L/(L + K_D)$.

This equation tells, that within a concentration range of ligand from 0.1-fold to 10-fold the K_D-value, B will move from 9.09% to 90.9% of B_{max}. In other words: Within two orders of magnitude around the half-maximally saturating amount of ligand concentration (the K_D-value) bound covers 81% of the total receptor sites. If less than two orders of magnitude are covered by the concentration range of radioligand used, or if the range is not distributed symmetrically around K_D, of course more than the residual 20% of not measured binding must be extrapolated for from the measured binding.

An example demonstrating the above discussed dependency of B on L is shown in Fig. 1C for ^3H-N-methylscopolamine binding to rat parotid gland membranes.

In binding studies usually more than one site is labeled due to additional non receptor binding of the radioligand to lipids, proteins, filter material etc. This is exemplified in Fig. 1A, where two sets of binding data of the radioligand were measured: Total binding and binding in the presence of 100 to 1000-fold excess of non-labeled ligand, the socalled non specific binding (nsb). Evaluation of parameters from such data sets may either be carried out using the equation (1) which is the generalization of equation (4) in a simultaneous fitting procedure of specific as well as non specific binding parameters as done in Fig. 1A. Alternatively a one site binding isotherm can be achieved by subtracting nsb from total binding measurements as done in Fig. 1B and 1C. However, it should be borne in mind that experimental errors in both data sets thus are added.

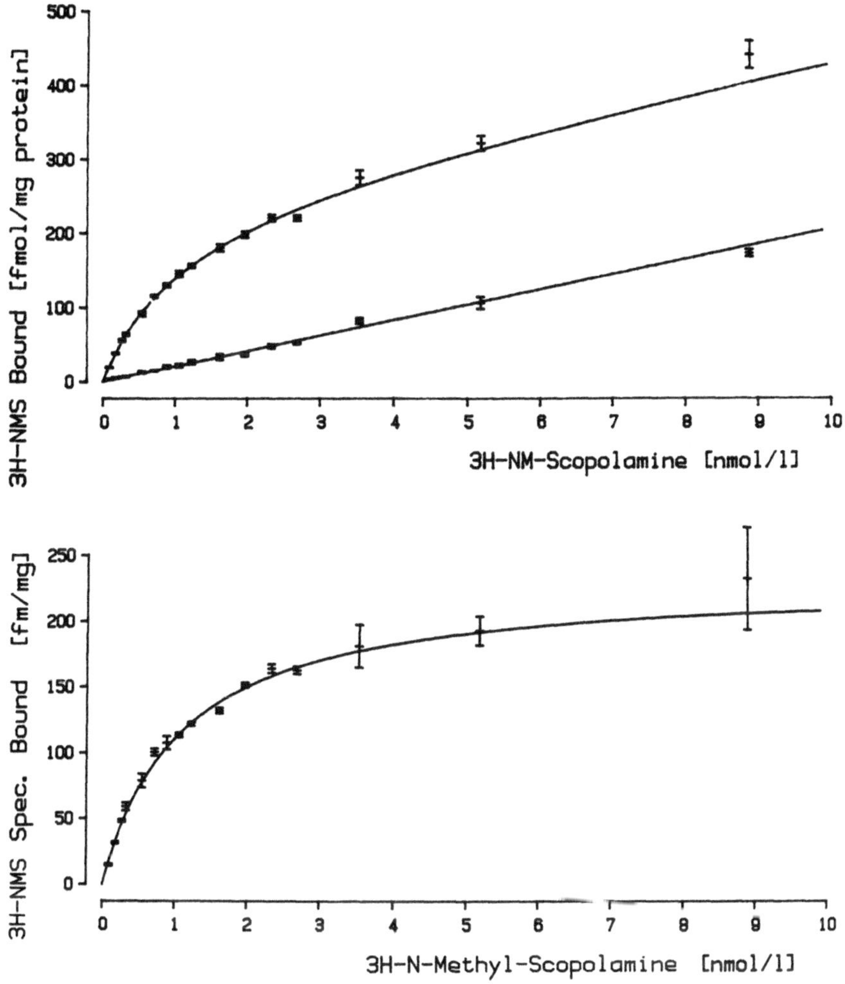

Fig. 1. Binding of ^{3}H-N-Methylscopolamine (^{3}H-NMS) to rat parotid gland membranes.
A. Total and non specific binding measurements (nsb, in the presence of 1 µmol/l scopolamine) and the binding function calculated for the data are presented. The bars refer to S.E.M. of the 6-fold replications of binding measurements.
B. Specific binding, linear/linear plot. nsb was subtracted from total binding measurements.

To get linearization of such a data set for linear regression analysis e.g. with a pocket calculator, enzymologists use plots of 1/B versus 1/L (Lineweaver-Burk plot) whereas in binding B/F versus B is preferred (Scatchard plot; F is free ligand concentration) for historical reasons. Unfortunately the Scatchard transformation projects errors in the experimental procedures inhomogeneously onto both axis which may result in strange deviations and has lead to some controversies (4,5). For this reason a non-linear analysis of untransformed data weighting each data pair according to the true experimental error of bound measurements should be preferred.

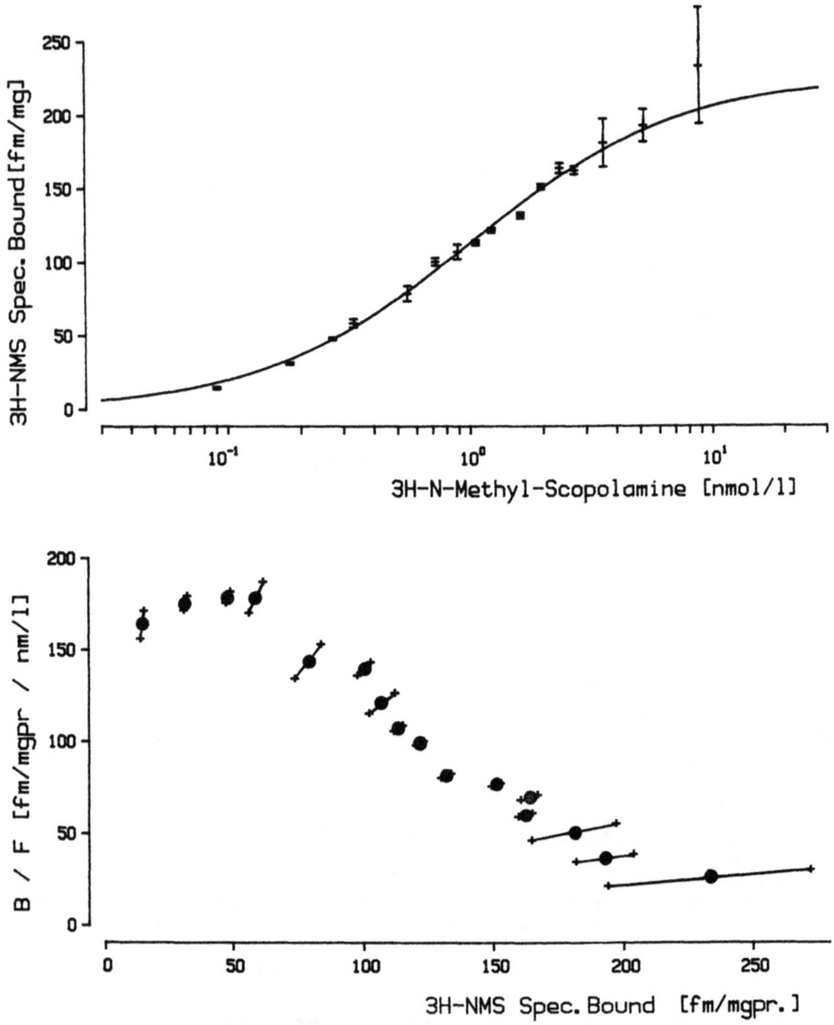

Fig. 1. (continued):
C. Specific binding, log/linear plot.
D. Scatchard transformation of specific binding measurements including S.E.M.

In cases of more than one binding site inherent in a data set (e.g. total binding in Fig. 1A) the Scatchard transformation anyhow yields curvilinearity and thus the only advantage of linear regression analysis – simplicity – is lost.

As shown in Fig. 1, non specific binding is superimposed onto specific binding to result in total binding thus comprising 2 binding sites. As can be seen from Fig. 2 any binding site has an initial slope of $\alpha = B_{max}/K_D$. If ligand concentrations of $\ll K_D$ are used, one may only achieve informations about this initial slope of a binding isotherm and state, that the range of ligand concentrations was not sufficient to demonstrate saturability. This situation is advantageous if a binding site is of non specific character. However a differentiating calculation of B_{max} and K_D

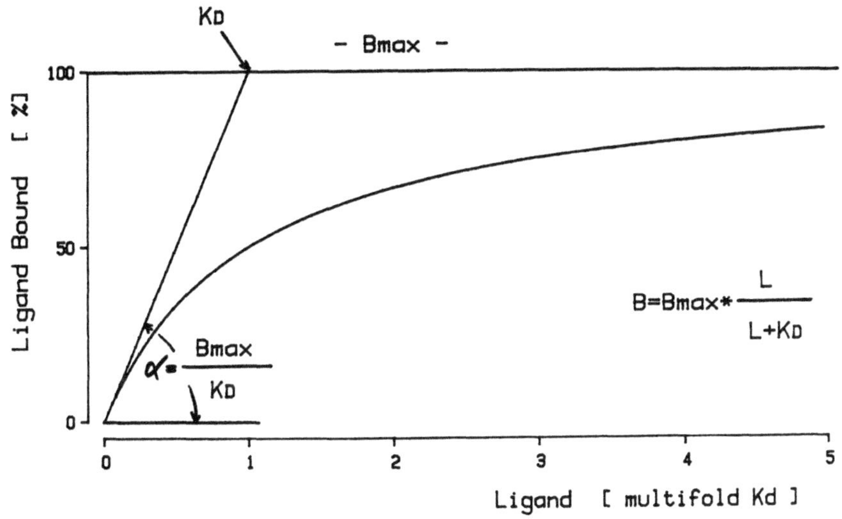

Fig. 2. Binding function at low ligand concentrations. The function describing binding at low ligand concentrations ($\ll K_D$) collapses to a straight line with intercept at the offset of the axes and a slope of $B_{max}/K_D = \alpha$.

of a specific binding site can neither be performed in this case. Fig. 3 shows an example of this situation:

The data used in the plot presented in Fig. 3 were kindly provided by Dr. Erdmann and his coworkers and show binding of ^{3}H-ouabain to rat heart membranes (for details, see 2).

This data set clearly shows two specific binding sites: One of high affinity ($K_D \sim 200$ pmol/2 ml) and a low affinity site for which only the ratio of B_{max}/K_D can be stated ($\sim 3 \times 10^{-4}$) indicating a K_D-value certainly beyond 5 nmol/2 ml (i.e. beyond the concentration range covered). Presenting this data set as originally measured (Fig. 3 B; c.f. 2) shows that the low affinity site is labeled by about 20 % of ^{3}H-ouabain bound and that the non-labeled ouabain does not compete for this second site to a significant extent within the range of concentrations covered. One possibility to measure such a low affinity site is the use of higher concentrations of ^{3}H-ligand thus labeling a larger portion of the low affinity site and to extend the range of concentrations of non labeled competitor.

Finally the kinetic approach to characterize two binding sites may be helpful. Using increasing concentrations of radioligand, increasing amounts of low affinity sites will be detectable in association and dissociation kinetics. Additionally, a differentiation between two non-cooperative separate binding sites from a cooperative one-site-site interaction is possible:

Inducing dissociation of bound radioligand via dilution of the samples and in parallel via displacement with excess of non-labelled ligand should yield the following informations:

(a) identical results from both approaches indicate non cooperative binding sites.

(b) Faster or slower dissociation reactions in displacement studies in comparison to dilution studies are indicative of negative or positive cooperative site-site interactions resp.

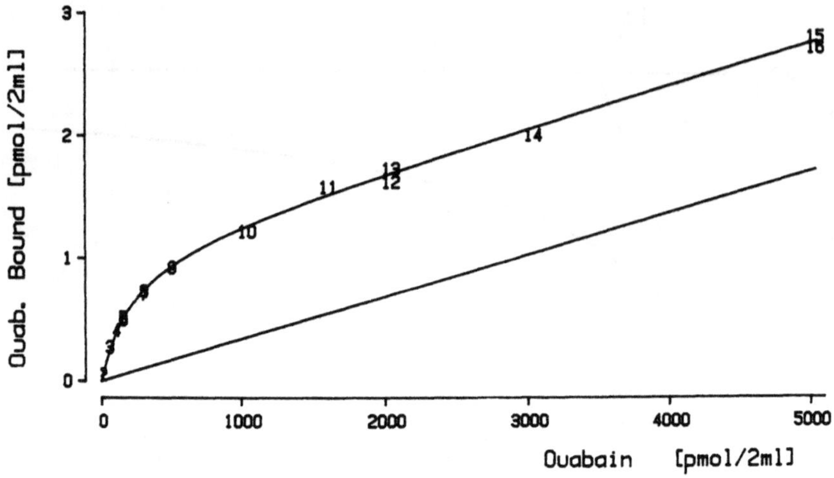

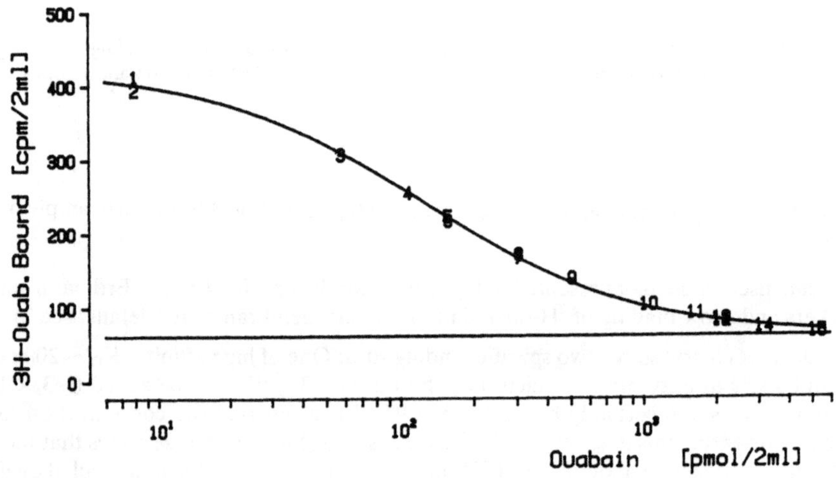

Fig. 3. Binding of ^{3}H-ouabain to rat heart membranes. For details of the method used, see (2).
A. The amount of ouabain bound is plotted versus the ouabain concentration (linear/linear) as a saturation isotherm.
B. The amount of ^{3}H-ouabain bound is plotted versus the ouabain concentration (log/linear) as a competition isotherm

Thus binding studies may truly give reliable information of ligand receptor interactions. However, these results should always be compared and even correlated with knowledge from independent investigations of pharmacological effects of the ligand and binding site preparation used. If no direct correlation between binding parameters and other pharmacological effects can be demonstrated, a revision of the design of binding experiments or a revision of the model explaining the role of the presumptive receptor site in the ligand/receptor / effector / effect cascade is necessary (1,2).

References

1. Brown L, Werdan K, Erdmann E (1983) Consequences of specific ^{3}H-ouabain binding to guinea pig left atria and cardiac cell membranes. Biochem Pharmacol 32:423–435
2. Erdmann E, Philipp G, Scholz H (1980) Cardiac glycoside receptor, (Na^{+} + K^{+}) ATPase activity and force of contraction in rat heart. Biochem Pharmacol 29:3219–3229
3. Feldman HA (1972) Mathematical theory of complex ligand-binding systems at equilibrium. Some methods for parameter fitting. Anal Biochem 48:317–338
4. Klotz IM (1983) Reply to: Number of receptor sites from Scatchard and Klotz graphs (Munson PJ, Rodbard D). Science 220:979–981
5. Munson PJ, Rodbard D (1983) Number of receptor sites from Scatchard and Klotz graphs: A constructive critique. Science 220:979–981
6. Scatchard G (1949): The attraction of proteins for small molecules and ions. N.Y. Acad Sci 51:660–672
7. Wiemer G, Wellstein A, Palm D, v. Hattingberg HM, Brockmeier D (1982) Properties of agonist binding at the β-adrenoceptor of the rat reticulocyte. Naunyn-Schmiedeberg's Arch Pharmacol 321:11–19
8. Williams LT, Lefkowitz RJ (1978) Receptor binding studies in adrenergic pharmacology (Raven Press, New York) pp 27–126

Authors' address:

Dr. A. Wellstein, Z. Pharmakologie, Klinikum der J. W. Goethe Universität, Theodor-Stern-Kai 7, 6000 Frankfurt/M.-70

Cardiac Glycosides and sodium/potassium-ATPase

K. Greeff and Alanna A. L. Fox

Institut für Pharmakologie, Universität Düsseldorf, Düsseldorf (FRG)

Summary

The sodium/potassium-ATPase complex is, according to modern research, the binding site for cardiac glycosides on the outer surface of the cell membrane and their receptor. Inhibition of this enzyme by cardiac glycosides leads for instance in the heart to a decrease or a delay in membrane sodium/potassium-ion transport, and indirectly to an increase in the intracellular ionized calcium-concentration and an increase in cardiac contractile force. According to recent observations the activity of the sodium/potassium-ATPase or its concentration, and therefore the concentration of binding sites can increase in some tissues after long term treatment with cardiac glycosides. This might explain the occasionally observed tolerance to digitalis glycosides.

Key words: sodium/potassium-ATPase, cardiac glycosides, enzyme induction, erythrocytes

Introduction

From the historic point of view, two research workers contributed greatly to the clarification of transmembrane ion transport and the mode of action of digitalis glycosides: J. H. Schatzmann in Bern and J. Chr. Skou in Aarhus.

In 1953 Schatzmann published the results of his experiments on cold stored erythrocytes (1). He demonstrated that the active ionic transport could be completely prevented by the addition of 10^{-5} g/ml strophoside.

As the glycoside changed neither the oxygen consumption nor the rate of glycolysis of the erythrocytes, Schatzmann came to the conclusion that the inhibition of the ion transport was not caused by an inhibition of the energy producing metabolism, but was however due to a blockade of the sodium/potassium-pump.

We were able to confirm these results in the isolated retina of bull's eye. A 2 hour incubation at 4 °C led to a decrease in the potassium content and an increase in sodium content. By a further incubation of the retina for 30 minutes at 37 °C a complete restitution of the intracellular ionic content could be observed. Strophanthin and digitoxin caused a concentration-dependent inhibition of this sodium/potassium-transport (2).

In 1957 Skou discovered an ATP hydrolysing enzyme in homogenates of crab nerves; this enzyme was activated by sodium and potassium in the presence of magnesium. The sodium/potassium-activated ATPase could be inhibited by strophanthin. The basal magnesium-activated ATPase-activity remained however uninfluenced by this glycoside (3).

In later experiments, Skou and his co-workers were able to show that the same enzyme was present in erythrocytes, in brain, kidney and other tissues (4, 5).

The cold stored erythrocytes as used by Schatzmann (1) were repeatedly used as model for studying the effects of cardiac glycosides. Dunham and Glynn (6) in England, Post et al. in the U.S.A. (7) were able to show that the same concentrations of glycosides which inhibit the sodium and potassium-transport in erythrocytes also inhibit the sodium and potassium-activated ATPase. Repke and co-workers were able to find a sodium/potassium-activated

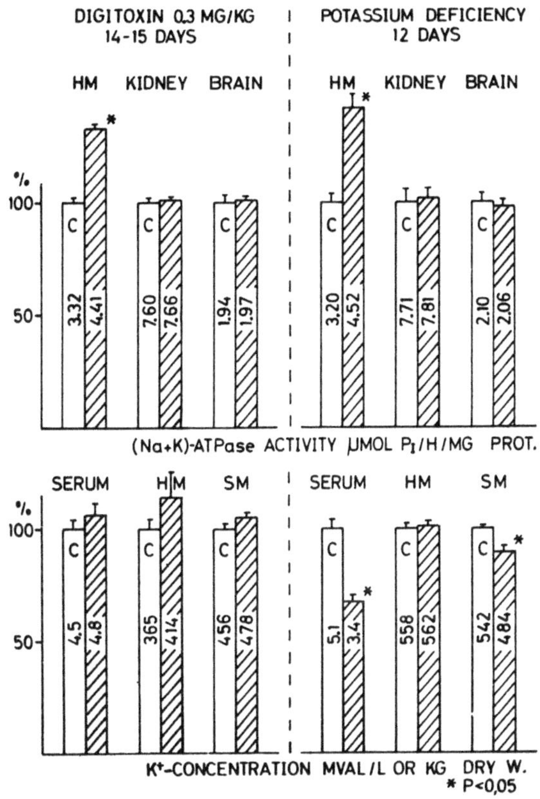

Fig. 1. Effect of digitoxin and K^+ deficient diet on the $(Na^+ + K^+)$-ATPase of the heart muscle (HM), kidney or brain of the guinea pig (upper graph) and on the K^+ concentration of serum, heart muscle (HM) or skeletal muscle (SM) (lower graph). Mean values and S.E.M. are shown for 4 enzymes prepared from 2–6 animals or K^+ concentrations of 6 animals. C = controls (20).

ATPase in cardiac muscle (8). They also made the observation that species dependent differences in the potency of digitalis glycosides were correlated with the sensitivity of the sodium/potassium-ATPase in cardiac muscle (9). Repke in 1962 was the first to suggest that the sodium/potassium-ATPase could be the receptor for digitalis.

In 1962, we made the observation that the positive inotropic effect of strophanthin and other glycosides on isolated Langendorff perfused guinea-pig hearts was accompanied by a loss of potassium ions depending upon the glycoside concentration (10). A definite correlation existed between the positive inotropic effect and the potassium loss within therapeutic concentrations. It increased more steeply at toxic concentrations. We know today that it is not the potassium loss that is the reason for the inotropic effect but the accompanying increase in intracellular sodium. This in turn leads to an increase in the intracellular ionized calcium concentration as first shown by Klaus and Kuschinsky (11) and Lüllmann and Holland (12). This is the basis for the positive inotropic effect of cardiac glycosides (13).

The elevation in intracellular calcium content by increased intracellular sodium is not only due to an increase in calcium-influx (14) or liberation of sarcolemmal calcium (15) but also to a reduction or retardation in the calcium-uptake into sarcoplasmic reticulum and mitochondria of cardiac muscle (16).

The question as to whether the sodium/potassium-activated ATPase is the receptor and mediator of the positive inotropic therapeutic action of digitalis glycosides is still controversial (13, 17). Erdmann and co-workers (19) have carried out several investigations indicating that the sodium/potassium-ATPase could be the digitalis receptor:
1. the inhibition of sodium/potassium-ATPase in human cardiac cell membranes correlates with its binding to cardiac muscle and 2. a definite correlation exists between ouabain-binding and increase in force of contraction.

Similar to results concerning the adrenergic alpha- and beta-receptors, a discussion has been taken up in recent years as to whether an up and down regulation exists for the digitalis receptors. Erdmann (18) showed that potassium deficiency causes an increase in the activity of the sodium/potassium-activated ATPase in the heart muscle of guinea pigs.

We were able to confirm these results (20): In guinea pigs the potassium deficiency over 12 days led to an increase in the sodium/potassium-ATPase in the cardiac muscle but the ATPase of the kidney and brain remained unaffected (Fig. 1).

A digitoxin treatment over a period of 14–15 days also led to an increase in the ATPase-activity of cardiac muscle. This digitoxin treatment did not alter the potassium content of the serum and cannot therefore be explained by an indirect influence on the ATPase due to a potassium loss. The increase in sodium and potassium-ATPase is dependent on the duration of treatment. A treatment of at least 7–24 days led to a significant increase in the sodium/potassium-ATPase activity of the cardiac muscle of the guinea pig whereas a treatment up to 5 days was uneffective (22).

Our experimental results could not be confirmed by investigations on the dog by Ku et al. (21). They have been, however, confirmed by recent investigations on erythrocytes: Cumberbatch and co-workers (23) found in 1981 that the sodium/potassium-ATPase activity of human erythrocytes increased significantly by 41 % after 29 months' treatment with digoxin (Table

Table 1.

		control	after glycoside treatment	Δ %	daily dose	duration months
		Na^+,K^+–ATPase activity				
1. Cumberbatch et al. (23)	human	5.1 ± 1.4$^{(A)}$	7.2 ± 2.2$^{(A)}$	+ 41	0.25 mg Digoxin	29
2. Fox et al. (unpublished)	guinea pigs	443 ± 63$^{(B)}$	624 ± 76$^{(B)}$	+ 41	70 μg/kg Ouabain	0.7
3. Wittacker et al. (24)	pigs	6.3 ± 0.2$^{(A)}$	10.2 ± 0.9$^{(A)}$	+ 62		3
		Ouabain binding capacity			17 μg/kg Digoxin	
	pigs	12.9 ± 1.7$^{(C)}$	19.4 ± 2.3$^{(C)}$	+ 50		3

Table 1. Effects of chronic cardiac glycoside treatment on Na^+,K^+-ATPase activity and ouabain binding capacity of erythrocytes.
1., 2. = S.D.; 3. = S.E.M.
(A) = $\mu molP_i \cdot g^{-1} \cdot Hb \cdot h^{-1}$
(B) = $nmolP_i \cdot mg^{-1}$ prot.$\cdot h^{-1}$
(C) = c.p.m.$\cdot 10^6$ cells

1). During this time, the potassium content of blood serum remained unchanged. Fox, Ingenhoven and Greeff (unpublished) have also found an increase of 41% in erythrocyte-ATPase of guinea pigs upon a 3 week treatment with ouabain (Table 1).

This year, Wittacker et al. (24) published results of an investigation in pigs. Here the erythrocyte-ATPase after 3 months treatment with digoxin increased from 6.3 to 10.2 μmol phosphate/g hemoglobin/hour, an increase of 62%. At the same time the ouabain-binding capacity increased by 50% (Table 1).

These experimental results led to the controversial question as to whether a pharmacological tolerance exists for cardiac glycosides. Ford et al. (25) investigated the influence of long-term digitoxin treatment on the rubidium-uptake of erythrocytes and came to the conclusion that a tolerance may develop. Guz and McHaffie postulate that the positive inotropic effect of digoxin in humans becomes weaker upon prolonged therapy (26). This is in accordance with the observation that upon withdrawal of digitalis glycoside many patients show no signs of cardiac failure (26, 27).

References

1. Schatzmann HJ (1953) Herzglykoside als Hemmstoffe für den aktiven Kalium- und Natriumtransport durch die Erythrocytenmembran. Helv Physiol Pharmacol Acta 11:346
2. Greeff K (1960) Über den Mechanismus der Wirkung von Digitalisglykosiden auf den Elektrolytstoffwechsel (Untersuchungen an der isolierten Retina). Verh Dtsch Ges Kreislaufforsch 26:127
3. Skou JChr (1957) The influence of some cations on an adenosine triphosphatase from peripheral nerves. Biochim Biophys Acta 23:394
4. Skou, JChr (1962) Preparation from mammalian brain and kidney of the enzyme system involved in active transport of Na^+ and K^+. Biochim Biophys Acta 58:314
5. Skou JChr (1960) The relationship of a (Mg^{2+} + Na^+)-activated, K^+-stimulated enzyme or enzyme system to the active, linked transport of Na^+ and K^+ across the cell membrane. Symposium on Membrane Transport and Metabolism, Prague, p. 228
6. Dunham ET, Glynn IM (1961) Adenosinetriphosphatase activity and the active movements of alkali metal ions. J Physiol 156:274
7. Post RL, Merritt CR, Kinsolving CR, Albright CD (1960) Membrane adenosine triphosphatase as a participant in the active transport of sodium and potassium in the human erythrocyte. J Biol Chem 235:1796
8. Repke K, Portius HJ (1963) Über die Identität der Ionenpumpen-ATPase in der Zellmembran des Herzmuskels mit einem Digitalis-Rezeptorenzym. Experientia 19:452
9. Repke K, Est M, Portius HJ (1965) Über die Ursache der Speciesunterschiede in der Digitalisempfindlichkeit. Biochem Pharmacol 14:1785
10. Greeff K, Meng K, Moog E (1962) Der Einfluß nichttoxischer und toxischer Konzentrationen herzwirksamer Glykoside auf die Kaliumbilanz isolierter Herzpräparate. Naunyn-Schmiedeberg's Arch Pharmacol 244:270
11. Klaus W, Kuschinsky G (1962) Über die Wirkung von Digitoxigenin auf den zellulären Ca-Umsatz im Herzmuskelgewebe. Naunyn-Schmiedeberg's Arch Pharmacol 244:237
12. Lüllmann H, Holland WC (1962) Influence of ouabain on an exchangeable calcium fraction, contractile force and resting tension of guinea-pig atria. J Pharmacol exp Ther 137:186
13. Akera T (1981) Effects of cardiac glycosides on Na^+,K^+-ATPase. In: Cardiac Glycosides, K. Greeff (ed.), Handb exp Pharmacol 56/I: 287, Springer-Verlag Berlin, Heidelberg, New York
14. Langer GA, Serena SD (1970) Effects of strophanthidin upon contraction and ionic exchange in rabbit ventricular myocardium: Relation to control of active state. J Mol Cell Cardiol 1: 65
15. Lüllmann H, Peters T (1976) On the sarcolemmal site of action of cardiac glycosides. Recent advances in studies on cardiac structure and metabolism. In: The sarcolemma, PE Roy, NS Dhalla (eds.) 9:311, University Park Press, Baltimore

16. Dransfeld H, Greeff K, Schorn A, Ting BT (1969) Calcium uptake in mitochondria and vesicles of heart and skeletal muscle in presence of potassium, sodium, k-strophanthin and pentobarbital. Biochem Pharmacol 18:1335
17. Godfraind, T.: Stimulation and inhibition of the Na^+,K^+– pump by cardiac glycosides. In: Cardiac Glycosides, K. Greeff (ed.), Handb exp Pharmacol 56/I:381, Springer-Verlag Berlin, Heidelberg, New York
18. Erdmann E (1981) Influence of cardiac glycosides on their receptor. In: Cardiac Glycosides, K. Greeff (ed.), Handb exp Pharmacol 56/I:337, Springer-Verlag Berlin, Heidelberg, New York
19. Erdmann E, Bolte HD, Lüderitz B (1971) The (Na^++K^+)-ATPase activity of guinea pig heart muscle in potassium deficiency. Arch Biochem Biophys 145:121
20. Bluschke V, Bonn R, Greeff K (1976) Increase in the (Na^++K^+)-ATPase activity in heart muscle after chronic treatment with digitoxin or potassium deficient diet. Eur J Pharmacol 37:189
21. Ku DD, Akera T, Brody TM, Weaver LC (1977) Chronic digoxin treatment on canine myocardial Na^+,K^+-ATPase. Naunyn-Schmiedeberg's Arch Pharmacol 301:39
22. Bonn R, Greeff K (1978) The effect of chronic administration of digitoxin on the activity of the myocardial (Na+K)-ATPase in guinea-pigs. Arch Int Pharmacodyn Therap 233:53
23. Cumberbatch M, Zareian K, Davidson C, Morgan DB, Swaminathan R (1981) The early and late effects of digoxin treatment on the sodium transport, sodium content and Na^++K^+-ATPase of erythrocytes. Br J Clin Pharmac 11:565
24. Wittacker J, Hawkins M, Swaminathan R (1983) Changes in erythrocyte sodium, sodium transport and ^3H ouabain binding capacity during digoxin administration in the pig. Life Sci 32:747
25. Ford AR, Aronson JK, Grahame-Smith DG, Carver JG (1979) The acute changes seen in cardiac glycoside receptor sites, ^{86}Rubidium uptake and intracellular sodium concentrations in the erythrocytes of patients during the early phases of digoxin therapy are not found during chronic therapy: pharmacological and therapeutic implications for chronic digoxin therapy. Br J Clin Pharmac 8:135
26. Guz A, McHaffie D (1978) The use of digitalis glycosides in sinus rhythm Clin Sci Mol Med 55:417
27. Bomann K, Allgulander S, Skoglund M (1981) Is maintenance digoxin necessary in geriatric patients? Acta Med Scand 210:493

Authors' address:

Prof. Dr. Kurt Greeff, Institut f. Pharmakologie, Universität Düsseldorf, Moorenstraße 5, 4000 Düsseldorf 1

Two receptors for cardiac glycosides in the heart

E. Erdmann, L. Brown, and K. Werdan

Medizinische Klinik I, Klinikum Großhadern, München (FRG)

Summary

Specific binding of ^{3}H-ouabain to rat cardiac cell membranes revealed a high affinity and a low affinity site. In order to test the pharmacological significance of these different types of binding sites, specific ^{3}H-ouabain binding, force of contraction and $^{86}Rb^+$-uptake were measured simultaneously in contracting cat papillary muscles and in guinea pig atria.

The results in the digitalis sensitive cat shows one type of cardiac glycoside receptors with high affinity ($K_D \sim 10^{-7}$M) for ouabain. The occupation of this receptor runs parallel with an increase in force of contraction and an inhibition of $^{86}Rb^+$-uptake. In the rather digitalis insensitive guinea pig, ^{3}H-ouabain binding also runs parallel with increased force of contraction, $^{86}Rb^+$-uptake, however, is only inhibited at toxic glycoside concentrations. Thus, in rat and guinea pig heart there exist at least two different digitalis receptors – the high affinity receptor seems to be coupled to inotropic effects, the low affinity receptor is linked to inhibition of (Na^++K^+)-ATPase.

Key words: ^{3}H-ouabain, cardiac glycoside receptors, (Na^++K^+)-ATPase, positive inotropy.

Introduction

(Na^++K^+)-ATPase, the enzyme system identified as the biochemical equivalent of the active transport system for Na^+ and K^+ across cell membranes, is specifically inhibited by cardiac glycosides (13). It has not been documented that the cardioactive steroids affect any other enzyme of the heart in the same low, clinically relevant concentrations. Thus, (Na^++K^+)-ATPase is supposed to be involved in the mechanism of action of cardiac glycosides (12).

Cardiac glycosides increase the force of contraction of the heart and they lead to cardiac arrhythmias, thereby having wanted, inotropic and unwanted, toxic effects, usually occurring only at higher concentrations. At present, most investigators agree that the toxic effects of cardiac glycosides are caused by an inhibition of the (Na^++K^+)-ATPase (1). There exists, however, quite a controversy in respect to the relationship between positive inotropy and activity of the enzyme (11). Is has been proposed that this enzyme – and thereby active cation transport – is stimulated, unaffected or inhibited by low but positively inotropic concentrations of cardiac glycosides (see 11). With radioactively labelled ouabain or digoxin, it has become possible to investigate the specific binding of these drugs to isolated cardiac cell membranes and to beating heart preparations. Thus, the simultaneous measurement of cardiac glycoside binding to its receptor, of the activity of (Na^++K^+)-ATPase and of force of contraction in the same preparation should allow us to answer the following questions:

1. is the binding of cardiac glycosides related to inhibition or stimulation of (Na^++K^+)-ATPase?
2. is the binding of cardiac glycosides related to the increase in force of contraction?

Supported by the DFG

3. is the $(Na^+ + K^+)$-ATPase inhibited when increased force of contraction is measured?
4. is there evidence for different cardiac glycoside binding sites, possibly one type connected with positive inotropy and another type connected with toxicity?

At first glance it seems to be simple to answer these questions by the respective experiments. It is, however, not possible to measure $(Na^+ + K^+)$-ATPase activity in an intact cardiac preparation. Therefore, we and others have measured the ouabain sensitive $^{86}Rb^+$-uptake instead, which is supposed to represent a reliable measure of the active cation transport or of the $(Na^+ + K^+)$-ATPase (2).

The experimental methods have been described in detail in the following papers (3, 4, 5).

For the sake of brevity the methodology is not repeated here.

Results

Isolated cardiac cell membranes

When investigating the specific ouabain binding to isolated cardiac cell membranes and the activity of the $(Na^+ + K^+)$-ATPase at the same time at various ouabain concentrations, we found an important discrepancy between these two parameters and between different species. Ouabain binding and a concomitant $(Na^+ + K^+)$-ATPase inhibition were measured in human, cat, beef, sheep and dog heart. This means that 50% of ouabain binding sites were occupied when 50% of total $(Na^+ + K^+)$-ATPase activity was inhibited (5). In rat, guinea pig and frog, however, we detected some specific ouabain binding without a measurable inhibition of the enzyme. $(Na^+ + K^+)$-ATPase was inhibited only by high ouabain concentrations. Thus, there is a discrepancy in these animal species between cardiac glycoside binding and $(Na^+ + K^+)$-ATPase inhibition (4). Rat cardiac cell membranes exhibit two different ouabain binding sites: a high affinity site ($K_D \sim 10^{-7}$M) and a low affinity site ($K_D \sim 10^{-5}$M). The $(Na^+ + K^+)$-ATPase is half maximally inhibited by 10^{-5}–10^{-4} M ouabain. Thus, it is suggested that the low affinity ouabain binding site is connected with the enzyme inhibition. The question remains, what is the function of the high affinity site?

Ouabain binding, $^{86}Rb^+$-uptake and force of contraction

The above mentioned experiments were performed in isolated cardiac cell membranes i.e. after destroying the cells. It is obvious, that an intact cardiac preparation might have different properties than cell membranes. Therefore, we have prepared rat ventricular slices (4), cat papillary muscles (6), and guinea pig left atria (3) in order to study this problem in intact tissue.

In cat papillary muscles the specific ^3H-ouabain binding to its binding sites goes along with an increase in force of contraction (Fig. 1). Ouabain sensitive $^{86}Rb^+$-uptake is measured as inhibited, when force of contraction is increased. Thus, in the digitalis sensitive cat, specific ouabain binding, increase in force of contraction and decrease in active cation transport run in parallel. Certainly, this finding does not mean that the inhibition of $(Na^+ + K^+)$-ATPase is the cause of increased force of contraction but at least the parameters measured are concomitant.

In rat ventricular slices and in guinea pig left atria (Fig. 2), again specific ouabain binding and force of contraction increased concomitantly. However, $^{86}Rb^+$-uptake was not inhibited by positive inotropic ouabain concentrations. Only when toxicity was regularly found, could we measure an inhibition of $^{86}Rb^+$-uptake. Looking at the ^3H-ouabain binding curves, it is obvious that the amount of tissue-bound ouabain increases beyond the point giving maximal positive inotropic response. This part of the binding curve goes along with the measured inhibition of $^{86}Rb^+$-uptake (and toxicity). Thus, our experimental data suggest a second, low

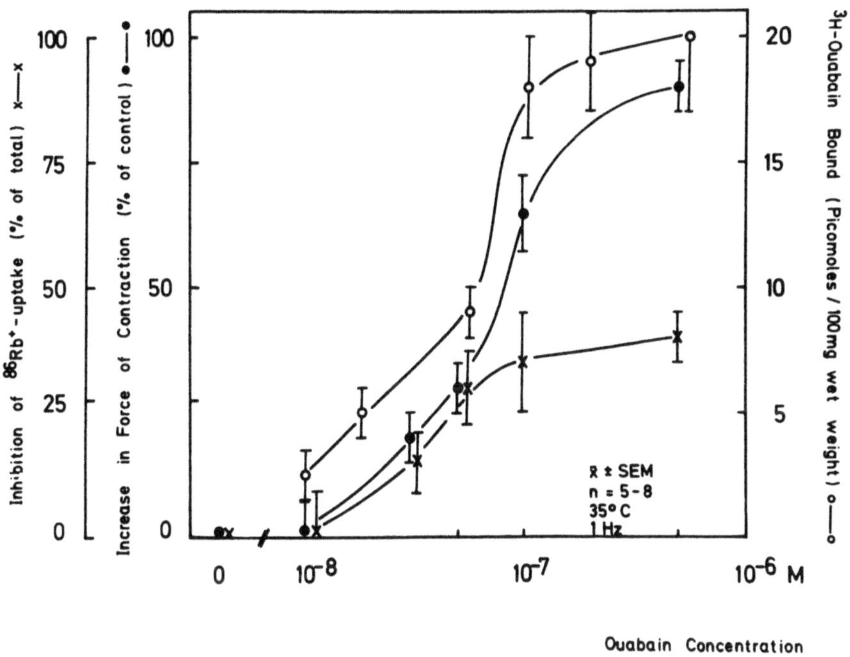

Fig. 1. Ouabain binding, force of contraction, and $^{86}Rb^+$-uptake in electrically stimulated contracting cat papillary muscles. The experiments were performed essentially as with rat ventricular strips (4).
This figure demonstrates a coincidence between ^{3}H-ouabain binding and increase in force of contraction as well as inhibition of active cation transport.

affinity ouabain binding site which may be responsible for the inhibition of the $(Na^+ + K^+)$-ATPase and possibly for signs of toxicity in rat and guinea pig heart.

Interestingly, the low affinity ouabain binding site is also found in isolated rat cardiac cell membranes ($K_D \sim 10^{-5}$–10^{-4}M). Therefore, the inhibition of $(Na^+ + K^+)$-ATPase in cell membranes and of $^{86}Rb^+$ uptake in intact cardiac tissue occurring at the same ouabain concentrations seem to be related to binding to the same site.

Under all conditions tested so far, at low concentrations ouabain binding to intact cardiac tissue was concomitant with increased force of contraction. If the two measured parameters (amount of ouabain bound and extent of increased force) were expressed as % of maximal, the two curves coincided. In the less digitalis sensitive species rat and guinea pig, a second, low affinity ouabain binding site was detected. This site was occupied by high ouabain concentrations only and was apparently connected with toxicity. In this case, a separation between positive inotropic and arrhythmogenic effects of cardiac glycosides appears to be possible, for instance by a drug with different affinities for each of the two receptors. In the highly digitalis sensitive species toxicity occurs slowly, as positive inotropy increases. In this case there is no distinction between the two modes of action of cardiac glycosides.

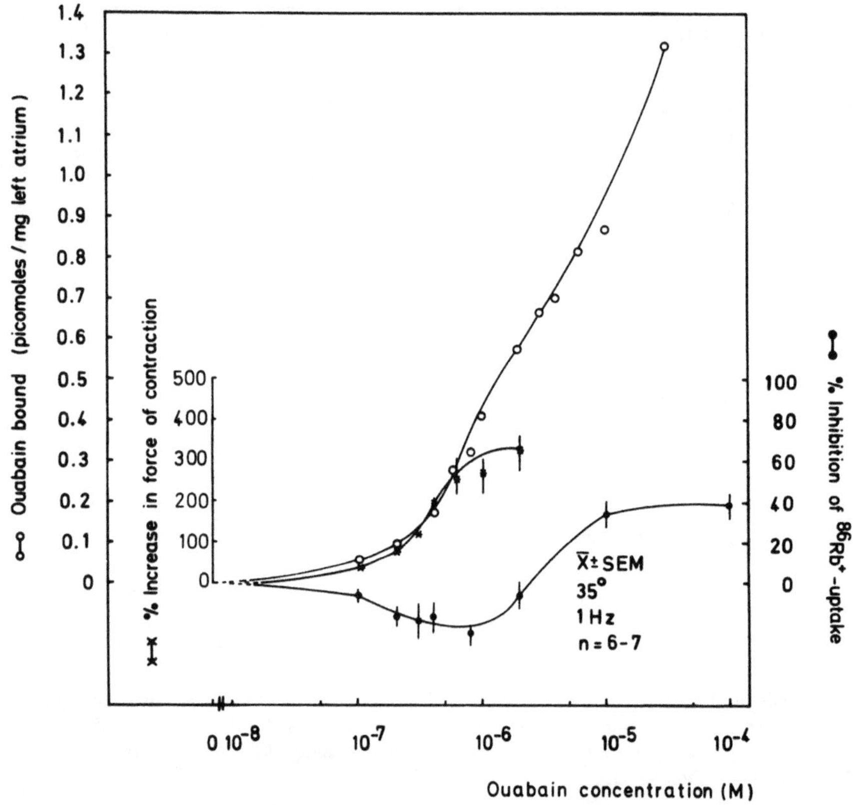

Fig. 2. Ouabain binding, force of contraction, and $^{86}Rb^+$-uptake in electrically stimulated guinea pig atria.
The experiments were performed essentially as in fig. 1 (for experimental details see 3).
This figure demonstrates a coincidence between specific ^{3}H-ouabain binding and increase in force of contraction. Active cation transport is not inhibited by positive inotropic ouabain concentrations, however.

Conclusions

There are three simple possibilities for the coupling of ouabain binding to inhibition of monovalent cation transport and increase in force of contraction:

1. specific ouabain binding to its receptor in $(Na^+ + K^+)$-ATPase causes an inhibition of the enzyme in such a way that one molecule of ouabain bound results in one molecule of $(Na^+ + K^+)$-ATPase inhibited. This is a 1:1 relationship (Fig. 3a).
2. two or more ouabain molecules are needed to inhibit one $(Na^+ + K^+)$-ATPase molecules. This means that ouabain binds to $(Na^+ + K^+)$-ATPase and inhibits the enzyme but there is less inhibition of the enzyme than ouabain bound (Fig. 3b).
3. ouabain binds to two different types of receptors. A high affinity site is connected to the positive inotropy, a low affinity site is connected to inhibition of $(Na^+ + K^+)$-ATPase. Thus, it would be possible to measure ouabain binding (and positive inotropy) without inhibition of the enzyme (Fig. 3c).

Our experiments seem to indicate that in digitalis sensitive species (man, beef, cat etc.) there is a 1:1 relationship between ouabain binding and inhibition of the $(Na^{+}+K^{+})$-ATPase. This finding goes along with the experimental work of Michael et al. (10) and Lee and Dagostino (9). In this case $(Na^{+}+K^{+})$-ATPase activity will be found as inhibited at positive inotropic ouabain concentrations.

In less digitalis sensitive species, we think we have provided evidence for two different ouabain binding sites (possibility 3, Fig. 3c). A high affinity ouabain binding site is connected with increase in force of contraction but not with inhibition of active monovalent cation transport. A second, low affinity ouabain binding site is connected with inhibition of $(Na^{+}+K^{+})$-ATPase. Thus, there is increased force of contraction without inhibition of the enzyme. The experimental data are in agreement with the data of Ghysel – Burton and Godfraind (7) and Lechat et al. (8).

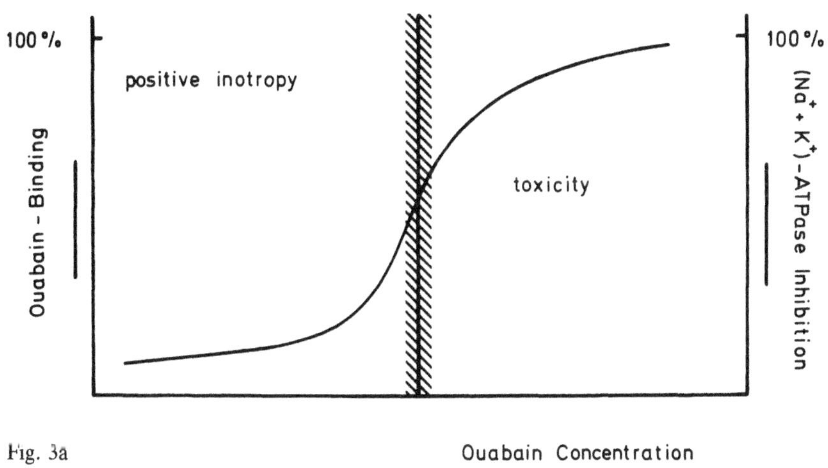

Fig. 3a

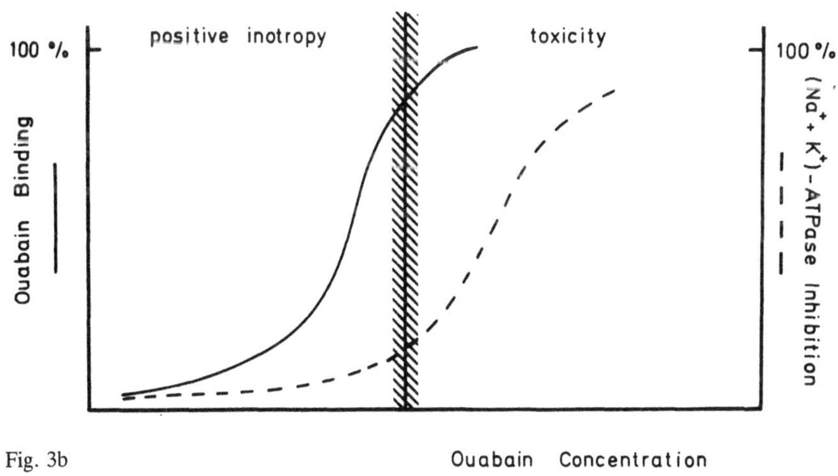

Fig. 3b

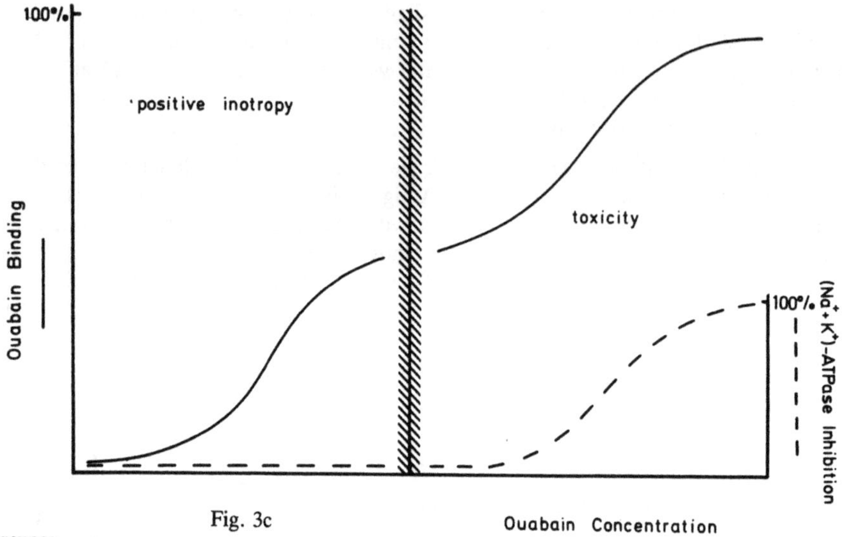

Fig. 3c

References

1. Akera T, Brody TM (1978) The Role of Na^+, K^+-ATPase in the Inotropic Action of Digitalis. Pharmacol Rev 29:187–219
2. Akera T, Yamamoto S, Temma K, Kim DH, Brody TM (1981) Is ouabain-sensitive rubidium or potassium uptake a measure of sodium pump activity in isolated cardiac muscle? Biochim Biophys Acta 640:779–790
3. Brown L, Werdan K, Erdmann E (1983) Consequences of specific ^{3}H-ouabain binding to guinea pig left atria and cardiac cell membranes. Biochem Pharmacol 32:423–435
4. Erdmann E, Philipp G, Scholz H (1980) Cardiac glycoside receptor, $(Na^+ + K^+)$-ATPase activity and force of contraction in rat heart. Biochem Pharmacol 29:3219–3229
5. Erdmann E Influence of cardiac glycosides on their receptor. in: Handbook of experimental pharmacology, Vol. 56/I by Springer-Verlag Berlin, Heidelberg, New York 1981
6. Erdmann E, Philipp G, Scholz H (1981) Evidence for two receptors for cardiac glycosides in the heart in: Cell membrane in function and dysfunction of vascular tissue. edit.: Godfraind T, Meyer P (Elsevier North-Holland, Amsterdam, New York, Oxford) 76–83
7. Ghysel-Burton J, Godfraind T (1979) Stimulation and inhibition of the sodium pump by cardioactive steroids in relation to their binding sites and their inotropic effect on guinea-pig isolated atria. Br J Pharmac 66:175–184
8. Lechat P, Malloy CR, Smith TW (1983) Active transport and inotropic state in guinea pig left atrium. Circ Res 52:411–422
9. Lee CO, Dagostino M (1982) Effect of strophanthidin on intracellular na ion activity and twitch tension of constantly driven canine cardiac purkinje fibers. Biophys J 40:185–198
10. Michael L, Schwartz A, Wallick E (1979) Nature of the transport adenosine triphosphatase digitalis complex: XIV. Inotropy and cardiac glycoside interaction with Na^+,K^+-ATPase of isolated cat papillary muscles. Molec Pharmacol 16:135–146
11. Noble D (1980) Mechanism of action of therapeutic levels of cardiac glycosides. Cardiovasc Res 14:495–514
12. Schwartz A (1976) Sodium – potassium adenosine triphosphatase – a receptor for digitalis? Biochem Pharmacol 25:237–239
13. Skou JC (1965) Enzymatic basis for active transport of Na^+ and K^+ across cell membrane. Rev Physiol 45:596–617

Authors' address:

Dr. E. Erdmann, Medizinische Klinik I der Universität Klinikum Großhadern, Marchioninistr. 15, 8000 München 70

Subclassification of cardiac glycoside receptors

T. Godfraind

Laboratoire de Pharmacodynamie Générale et de Pharmacologie, Université Catholique de Louvain, Bruxelles (Belgium)

Key words: cardiac glycosides, glycoside receptors, $(Na^{+}+K^{+})$-ATPase, positive inotropy, receptor-binding.

Introduction

It is widely accepted that cardiac glycosides are therapeutically efficient to treat heart failure. Their beneficial action may be attributed to their positive inotropic effect, even if their action on preload and afterload has to be taken into account (12). Despite of the large interest devoted to these drugs, the mechanism of their inotropic action is still a matter of controversy. In 1953, Schatzman reported that cardiac glycosides inhibit the ionic restoration of red blood cells occurring during rewarming after an incubation at low temperature which altered the physiological distribution of Na and K. This observation showed that the glycosides alter the transport of monovalent cations against their electrochemical gradient. In 1957, Skou discovered Na,K-ATPase and since, the mechanism of Na and K transport has been extensively investigated. Several physiological processes are coupled to the Na,K-pump, the identification of this coupling has been demonstrated by blockade of the pump by large doses of cardiac glycosides.

Repke (30) has proposed that the positive inotropic effect of cardiac glycosides was directly related to the inhibition of the Na,K-pump. This hypothesis has been further developed by Langer who proposed that the Na-Ca exchange mechanism described by Reuter was the physiological mechanism involved in the inotropic action of ouabain (25; 31).

However, not all the actions of cardiac glycosides can be attributed to Na,K-pump inhibition and several observations show that at low doses, cardiac glycosides stimulate the pump (15). Furthermore, it has been proposed that their positive inotropic effect could be the sum of two processes: the inhibition of the pump and a still unknown mechanism (18; 23; 28).

In this report, I would like to show that the complex action of cardiac glycosides could be due to the heterogeneity of their binding sites and to the interaction of glycosides with an endogenous digitalis-like factor. Furthermore, a comparative study of the actions of cardioactive steroids in relation to their structure shows differences in their pharmacological profile (this is namely the case for ouabain and dihydroouabain). The use of the classical concepts of agonism and antagonism allows an adequate characterization of the differences in pharmacological profile.

The binding of cardiac glycosides to their receptors

The binding of cardiac glycosides to their receptors has been studied using intact tissues or microsomal preparations (13). Identification of the binding of glycosides to microsomal fractions containing Na,K-ATPase has been initiated by Matsui and Schwartz (27). Their study has been confirmed several times showing that the binding is influenced by the presence of various ligands: ATP, Na, K, Mg. The enzyme phosphorylation increased the affinity of the enzyme for ouabain. According to the ligands supporting the binding, two types of complexes have been proposed to exist. Binding to type I (formed in the presence of Mg and ATP) is enhanced by Na. Binding to type II (formed in the presence of Mg and Pi) is antagonized by Na. Binding to both complexes is antagonized by K (2).

Studies of a large number of natural or semisynthetic compounds have shown that the 3β-sugar and the 17β-lactone ring are involved in glycoside binding to Na,K-ATPase. According to Yoda, the binding of the steroid moiety precedes the sugar binding and induces a receptor conformational change that allows pseudo-irreversible binding of the sugar. The unsaturated lactone ring is regarded as a most essential pharmacodynamic group. According to the model proposed by Thomas et al. (34), the unsaturated lactone ring could bind to a two points attachment. This would be facilitated by a resonance in the ring allowing positive charges in C_{20} and negative ones on the carbonyl group. Such a resonance does not occur when the lactone ring is saturated giving dihydroouabain. An electrostatic binding between C_{20} of the unsaturated lactone and a putative negative charge of the receptor would not occur with the dihydroderivatives which would only be bound through a hydrogen bond. The qualitative differences between ouabain and dihydroouabain that will be summarized below are consistent with these chemical differences. Although the first studies (7) reported only the existence of one class of binding sites, the existence of a second high affinity receptor was postulated by Godfraind (13) to account for the "low-dose" effect in the heart (and see below). Studies now reported with various microsomal preparations support the concept of the heterogeneity of cardiac glycoside binding sites. A similar conclusion may be drawn from studies with intact heart from various species and as recently demonstrated, with isolated myocytes from rat heart (for ref. see 9).

As Fig. 1 illustrates for the guinea-pig atria, a high affinity, low capacity binding of ouabain has been identified in the nanomolar range and a low affinity high capacity binding can be identified in a concentration range 2 or 3 orders of magnitude higher (16).

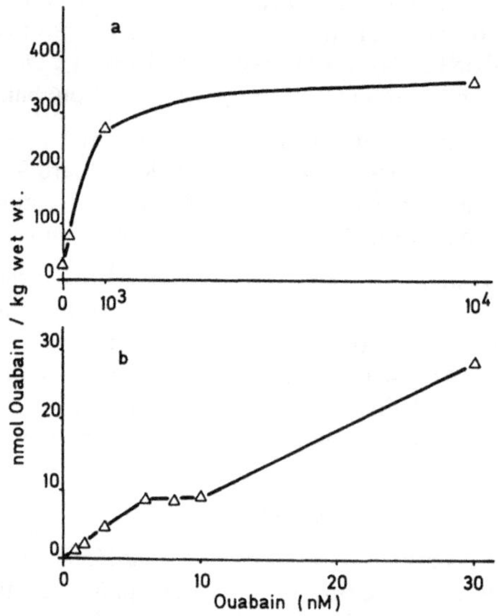

Fig. 1. Specific binding of ouabain to isolated guinea-pig atria as a function of glycoside concentration a) saturable binding to low affinity sites; b) saturable binding to high affinity sites. Note that the range of concentrations between a) and b) is of 2 orders of magnitude (16).

The high affinity binding sites represent 5 to 10 per cent of the total number of sites. This figure could at glance appear to be very low, but it corresponds to about 10^4 molecules bound per cardiac cell at maximum binding to high affinity sites.

There are several experimental arguments suggesting that high and low affinity binding sites are related to two Na, K-ATPases. In both guinea-pig (20) and rat (29) microsomes, the ligands supporting the binding of ouabain are the same. In rat heart microsomes, the existence of two different Na, K-ATPase inhibitory processes can be identified when a wide range of ouabain concentrations is studied. Noël and Godfraind have concluded that two Na, K-ATPase isozymes coexist in rat heart microsomes. The high and low affinity sites are in a ratio of 1 to 10. They have not only a difference in affinity for cardiac glycosides but also for KCl which, as mentioned above, reduces the affinity of Na, K-ATPase for ouabain. In guinea-pig (11) and in rat heart, this reduction is less pronounced for high than for low affinity sites as if the sites with the highest affinity for cardiac glycosides presented the lowest affinity for KCl. This explains why the delineation of two cardiac glycosides binding sites is more obvious in the presence of KCl. For a given species, the relative importance of the high and low affinity binding sites may vary according to the anatomical part of the heart. Rat heart ventricles contain more high affinity binding sites than rat atria (9). Furthermore, the affinity ratio between the high and low affinity sites may be different in different species, for example, taking ouabain as a ligand, it is equal to 60–70 in rat heart microsomes and only to 7 in human heart microsomes (6; 9).

The action of cardiac glycosides on the Na, K-pump in isolated heart

Schatzman's observation that cardiac glycosides inhibit the active transport of monovalent cations in red blood cells has been extended to a wide variety of tissues including heart (13).

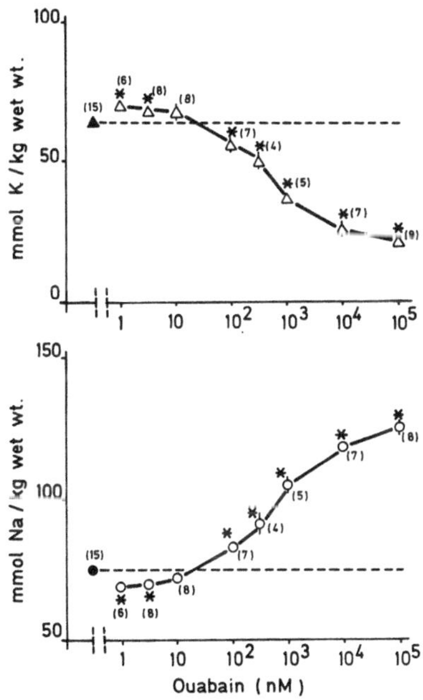

Fig. 2. (a) Potassium and (b) sodium content of stimulated left atria from guinea-pig incubated at 30° C for 3 h in various concentrations of ouabain. The number of determinations at each point is indicated in brackets. Note increased gradient in the low range (10^{-9} to 10^{-8} M) and decreased gradient in the higher range (> 10^{-8} M) (16).

We have examined the action of ouabain dosages varying from 10^{-9} M to 10^{-3} M on the ionic composition of guinea-pig isolated left atria stimulated at 3.3 Hz. The dosage range for cardiac glycosides action is dependent upon the concentration of KCl in the medium: lowering KCl does shift to the left this range and increasing KCl does shift it to the right (11). Figure 2 illustrates an experiment performed with 6 mM KCl in the medium (16). It shows that high doses of ouabain ($>10^{-7}$ M) increase the Na content and decrease the K content of the tissue. This reduction in ionic gradients may be attributed to the inhibition of the Na-K pump. Low doses of ouabain ($>10^{-8}$ M) produce an opposite effect since the Na content decreases and the K content increases. This increase in ionic gradients has been attributed to the stimulation of the Na-K pump. Studies using ^{42}K as an index of the activity of the Na-K pump have allowed to confirm these observations (11; 17; 24). One of the characteristics of the ouabain-evoked pump stimulation is to be transient. This has namely been documented with digoxin by Godfraind and Ghysel-Burton (17) who have shown that in guinea-pig atria incubated at 30° C, digoxin 10^{-8} M evoked a large stimulation of ^{42}K uptake after 45 min incubation but an inhibition after 3 hrs incubation. Observation of the ouabain-evoked stimulation of ^{42}K uptake is consistent with electrophysiological measurements of the reversal potential iK_2 (4) and with the observation that α_i decreases in sheep Purkinje fibres treated by low doses of cardiac glycosides (5). The unsaturation of the lactone ring is required to observe Na, K-pump stimulation by cardiac glycosides: dihydroouabain is 80 times less potent than ouabain for inhibition but does not stimulate the pump (11). The observations on intact tissue are difficult to reconcile with those on purified Na, K-ATPase. Indeed, concentrations of glycosides which stimulate the pump are slightly inhibitory on guinea-pig heart Na, K-ATPase preparations. To account for this, Godfraind (14) has proposed that the action of low doses of glycosides should be considered as a derepression rather than a true stimulation, postulating the existence of a specific endogenous repressor substance with which cardiac glycosides could compete. Recent studies show that a digoxin-like material can be found in various mammalian tissues. The nature of this factor that was called cardiodigin is still unknown (21). Information actually available shows that cardiodigin is very likely an endogenous factor (3), that it inhibits Na, K-ATPase and competes with ouabain binding. The interaction with Na, K-ATPase is dependent on KCl. Furthermore, cardiodigin has a specific reaction with digoxin antibodies. Hougen et al. (24) have shown that the stimulation of the pump by ouabain is blocked by large doses of propranolol and is absent after catecholamine depletion. They have concluded that endogenous catecholamines could be involved in pump stimulation. This conclusion does not rule out the possibility of interaction of glycosides with cardiodigin. Further experiments will certainly contribute to a better understanding of this mechanism.

The inotropic effect of cardiac glycosides and its antagonism by dihydroouabain

The contractility of cardiac muscle is largely controlled by intracellular Na concentration regulating transmembrane Ca translocation through Na-Ca exchange system (25; 31).

This mechanism allows to understand how the activity of the Na, K-pump affects cardiac contraction. Decrease in the activity of the pump that can be achieved by a decrease in extracellular KCl concentration evokes a positive inotropic effect resulting from increased intracellular activator Ca. On isolated strips of cardiac muscle, cardiac glycosides exert a powerful inotropic action. Repke (30) has proposed that it was entirely due to Na, K-ATPase inhibition and thereby to inhibition of the Na, K-pump. However, detailed analysis has shown that it is necessary to distinguish two concentration ranges in the inotropic effect of cardiac glycosides: a low and a high doses effect (13; 22; 23; 26; 28).

The dose-response curve of isolated heart preparations to cardiac glycosides is dependent on several factors including the cardiac glycoside used, the composition of the perfusion fluid, the rate of stimulation, the nature of the stimulating electrodes (field or needle), the

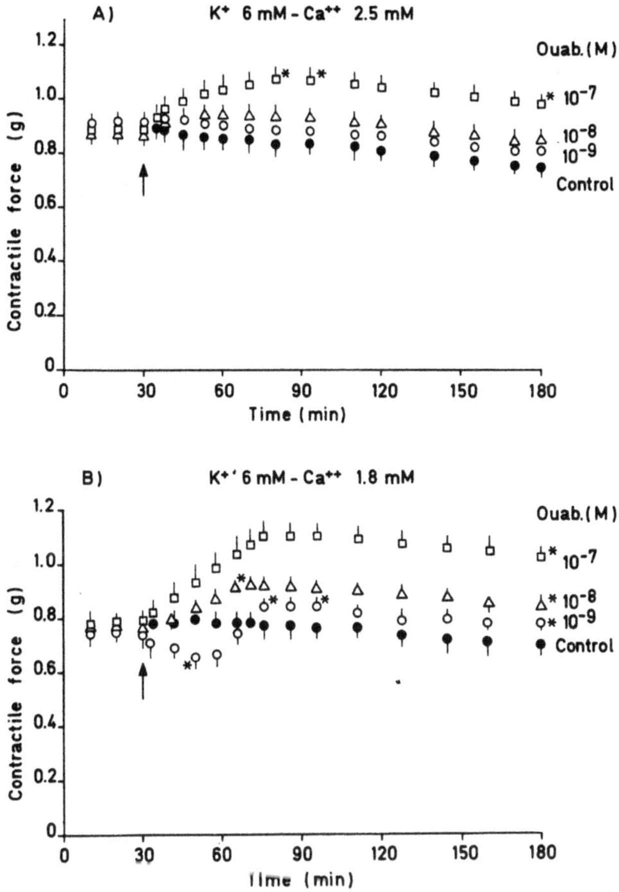

Fig. 3. Influence of $CaCl_2$ concentration on the inotropic effect of low doses of ouabain. Note the diphasic response to ouabain 10^{-9} M in B (22).

anatomical origin and the integrity of the preparation, its actual content in intrinsic neurotransmitters and the species from which it is dissected. This makes difficult the comparison between various authors if the experimental conditions are not identical. Figure 3 illustrates this complexicity, as it reports the inotropic effect of various concentrations of ouabain in isolated guinea-pig atria when the difference is just the concentration of calcium in the perfusate. It appears that the inotropic action of low doses of cardiac glycosides may be absent when the extracellular calcium concentration is above a certain level. It is also interesting to examine in Fig. 3 the inotropic response to ouabain 10^{-9} M as function of the time after the addition of the glycoside. Ouabain evokes a negative inotropic effect followed by a return to initial inotropy and by a positive effect. It is likely that in this experiment, the stimulation of the Na, K-pump by ouabain was of a sufficient intensity to initially counteract the inotropic action observable later on, because of the transient state of the stimulation. Experiments that have been conducted in various species: guinea-pig (11; 26), rat (1; 8; 9) and sheep Purkinje fibres (23) with dihydroouabain show that, by contrast to ouabain, there is no evidence for an inotropic effect independent from Na, K-pump inhibition (18). When the specific binding of 3H-ouabain is studied in the presence of increasing concentrations of ouabain or of dihydroouabain, there is a parallel displacement of the radioligand from its receptors, indicating that dihydroouabain can bind to all the sites where ouabain can be bound, and therefore to both high and low affinity sites (19). Following a classical pharmacological assumption, this means that the concepts of agonism and antagonism could be applied to the interaction of cardiac glycosides with the high affinity sites. Experiments with dihydroouabain done with guinea-pig and rat heart have allowed to observe that the glycosides with an saturated lactone ring are antagonists for the inotropic action of ouabain. Studies with rat isolated ventricles show that the antagonism is exerted at the level of the high affinity sites (9; 19).

In those experiments, the inotropic response to ouabain was reduced when dihydroouabain was added before the ouabain (Fig. 4). We have not been able to reverse ouabain inotropic effect once it was established. In this respect, the antagonism is not identical to a classical interaction of, for example, a β-stimulant with a β-blocker.

Concluding remarks

Recent experimental observations indicate that specific receptors for cardiac glycosides in heart muscle may be sub-classified into high and low affinity sites. The low affinity sites interact with glycosides to produce an inotropic effect that is related to increase in intracellular Na content and thereby to an interaction with Na-Ca exchange mechanism. The interaction of cardiac glycosides with the high affinity sites seems to present characteristics similar to those observed when an agonist interacts with its specific receptors. For such an interaction, the lactone ring appears to play a major role since its saturation yields to antagonistic properties. In addition, it could be that an endogenous digitalis-like factor could interfere with the pharmacological action of cardiac glycosides. This allows to understand the mechanism of

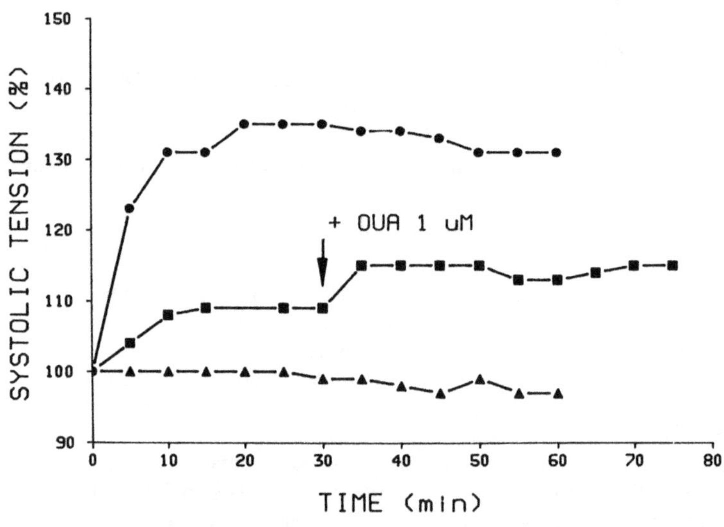

Fig. 4. Rat isolated ventricle, inotropic action of ouabain.
▲ Controls
● Response to ouabain 1 μM
■ Response to dihydroouabain 3 μM, then to ouabain 1 μM.
Note the reduction of ouabain response after dihydroouabain (9).

Na, K-pump stimulation. But more experimental work is needed to ascertain both the existence and the physiological role of such a factor.

References

1. Adams RJ, Schwartz A, Grupp G, Grupp IL, Lee, SW, Wallick ET, Powell T, Twist VW, Gathiram P (1982) High-affinity ouabain binding site and low-dose positive inotropic effect in rat myocardium. Nature 296:167–169
2. Akera T (1981) Effects of cardiac glycosides on (Na + K)-ATPase. In: Cardiac Glycosides, Handb. Exp Pharm Vol 56/I, pp 287–383, Greeff K (Ed) Springer-Verlag, Berlin Heidelberg New York
3. Castaneda H. G, Godfraind T (1984) Effect of high sodium intake on tissue distribution of endogenous digitalis-like material in the rat. Clin Sci 66:225–228
4. Cohen I, Daut J, Noble D (1976) An analysis on the action of low concentrations of ouabain on membrane currents in Purkinje fibres. J Physiol (London) 260:75–103
5. Deitmer JW, Ellis D (1970) The intracellular sodium activity of cardiac Purkinje fibres during inhibition and reactivation of the Na/K pump. J Physiol (London) 284:241–259
6. De Pover A., Godfraind T (1979) Interaction of ouabain with (Na + K)-ATPase from human heart and from guinea-pig heart. Biochem Pharmacol 28:3051–3056
7. Erdmann E, Schoner W (1973) Ouabain-receptor interactions in (Na + K)-ATPase preparations. II. Effect of cations and nucleotides on rate constants and dissociation constants. Biochim Biophys Acta 330:302–315
8. Erdmann E, Philipp G, Scholz H (1980) Cardiac glycoside receptor, (Na + K)-ATPase activity and force of contraction in rat heart. Biochem Pharmacol 29:3219–3229
9. Finet M, Godfraind T, Noël F (1983) The inotropic effect of ouabain and its antagonism by dihydroouabain in rat isolated atria and ventricles in relation to specific binding sites. Br J Pharmac 80:751–759
10. Ghysel-Burton J, Godfraind T (1977) High and low affinity ouabain binding sites in guinea-pig atria. Br J Pharmac 498P
11. Ghysel-Burton J, Godfraind T (1979) Stimulation and inhibition of the sodium pump by cardioactive steroids in relation to their binding sites and their inotropic effect on guinea-pig isolated atria. Br J Pharmac 66:175–184
12. Godfraind T (1973) The therapeutic mode of action of cardiac glycosides. Arch int Pharmacodyn Ther 206:384–388
13. Godfraind T (1975) Cardiac glycoside receptors in the heart. Biochem Pharmacol 24:823–827
14. Godfraind T (1980) Stimulation et inhibition de la pompe à sodium par les hétérosides cardiotoni ques. Bull Acad Roy Méd Belg 135:174–192
15. Godfraind T (1982) Stimulation and inhibition of the Na, K-pump by cardiac glycosides. In: "Cardiac Glycosides" Greef K Ed Handb. Exp Pharm, Vol 56/I, pp 381–393. Springer-Verlag, Berlin Heidelberg New York
16. Godfraind T, Ghysel-Burton J (1977) Binding sites related to ouabain-induced stimulation or inhibition of the sodium pump. Nature 265:165–166
17. Godfraind T, Ghysel-Burton J (1979) The cardioactive properties of SC4453, a digoxin analogue with a C17 β-pyridazine ring. Eur J Pharmacol 60:337–344
18. Godfraind T, Ghysel-Burton J (1980) Independence of the positive inotropic effect of ouabain from the inhibition of the heart Na/K pump. Proc Natl Acad Sci USA 77:3067–3069
19. Godfraind T, Ghysel-Burton J, De Pover A (1982) Dihydroouabain is an antagonist of ouabain inotropic action. Nature 299:824–826
20. Godfraind T, De Pover A, Tona Lutete D-N (1980) Identification with potassium and vanadate of two classes of specific ouabain binding sites in a (Na + K)-ATPase preparation from the guinea-pig heart. Biochem Pharmacol 29:1195–1199
21. Godfraind T, De Pover A, Castaneda Hernandez, Fagoo M (1982) Cardiodigin endogenous digitalis-like material from mammalian heart. Arch int Pharmacodyn Ther 258:165–167
22. Grupp G, Grupp IL, Ghysel-Burton J, Godfraind T, Schwartz A (1982) Effects of very low concentrations of ouabain on contractile force of isolated guinea-pig, rabbit and cat atria and right ventricular papillary muscles: an interinstitutional study. J Pharmacol Exp Ther 220:145–151

23. Hart G, Noble D, Shimoni Y (1983) The effects of low concentrations of cardiotonic steroids on membrane currents and tension in sheep Purkinje fibres. J Physiol (London) 334:103–131
24. Hougen TJ, Spicer N, Smith TW (1981) Stimulation of monovalent cation active transport by low concentrations of cardiac glycosides. Role of catecholamines. J Clin Invest 68:1207–1214
25. Langer GA (1983) The sodium pump lag revisited. J Mol Cell Cardiol 15:647–651
26. Lechat P, Mallory CR, Smith TW (1983) Active transport and inotropic state in guinea-pig left atrium. Circ Res 52:411–422
27. Matsui H, Schwartz A (1966) Kinetic analysis of ouabain-K and Na interaction on a Na, K-dependent adenosine triphosphatase from cardiac tissue. Biochem Biophys Res Commun 25:147–152
28. Noble D (1980) Mechanism of action of therapeutic levels of cardiac glycosides. Cardiovascular Res 14:495–514
29. Noël F, Godfraind T (1984) Heterogeneity of ouabain specific binding sites and (Na + K)-ATPase inhibition in microsomes from rat heart. Biochem Pharmacol, 33:47–53
30. Repke K (1963) Metabolism of cardiac glycosides. In: "Proceedings of the First International Pharmacological Meeting, Stockholm", Vol. III New Aspect of cardiac glycosides. Wilbrand W Ed pp 47–74 (Pergamon Press New York)
31. Reuter H (1974) Exchange of calcium ions in the mammalian myocardium. Mechanisms and physiological significance. Circ Res 34:599–605
32. Schatzmann HJ (1953) Herzglycoside als Hemmstoffe für den aktiven Kalium- und Natrium-Transport durch die Erythrocyten Membran. Helv Physiol Pharmacol Acta 11:346–354
33. Skou JC (1957) The influence of some cations on an adenosine triphosphatase from peripheral nerves. Biochim Biophys Acta 23:394–401
34. Thomas R, Allen J, Pitts BJR, Schwartz A (1979) Cardenolide analogs. An explanation for the unusual properties of AY 22241. Eur J Pharmacol 53:227–237
35. Yoda A (1973) Structure-activity relationships of cardiotonic steroids for the inhibition of sodium- and potassium-dependent adenosine triphosphatase. Dissociation rate constants of various enzyme – cardiac glycoside complexes formed in the presence of magnesium and phosphate. Mol Pharmacol 9:51–60

Author's address:

Prof. Dr. T. Godfraind, Lab. de Pharmacodynamie Générale et de Pharmacologie, Université Catholique de Louvain, U.C.L. 7350, Avenue Emmanuel Mounier, 73, B-1200 Bruxelles (Belgium)

Cardiac glycoside binding sites in cultured heart muscle cells

K. Werdan, B. Zwißler, B. Wagenknecht, W. Krawietz and E. Erdmann

Medizinische Klinik I der Universität München (FRG)

Summary

Binding of (^{3}H)-ouabain to cultured cardiac muscle and non muscle cells from chicken embryos and neonatal rats has been characterized and correlated with ouabain-induced inhibition of the sodium pump, as well as with the positive inotropic action of the drug.

1. Cardiac muscle and non muscle cells from 10–12 day-old chicken embryos are characterized by a single class of ouabain binding sites (muscle cells: dissociation constant $K_D = 1.5 \times 10^{-7}$M; binding capacity B = 2.6 pmoles/mg cell protein).

2. Two classes of ouabain binding sites, however, have been found in cardiac muscle and non muscle cells from 1–3 day-old, neonatal rats (muscle cells: high affinity, low capacity sites: $K_D = 3.2 \times 10^{-8}$M, B = 0.2 pmoles/mg protein; low affinity, high capacity sites: $K_D = 7.1 \times 10^{-6}$M, B = 2.6 pmoles/mg protein).

3. Half maximal inhibition of active ($^{86}Rb^+ + K^+$)-influx occurs at 5.8×10^{-7}M ouabain in chicken heart muscle cells and at 1.3×10^{-5}M in rat heart muscle cells ($[K^+]$ = 0,75 mM). Decreases in cell-K^+ ($EC_{50} = 6.7 \times 10^{-7}$M and 1.9×10^{-5}M) and increases in cell-Na^+ (7.4×10^{-7} and 10^{-5}–10^{-4}M) parallel ouabain-induced inhibition of the sodium pump.

4. Up to 10^{-6}M, ouabain does not affect velocity of cell wall motion in cultured rat heart muscle cells. A concentration-dependent increase in cell wall motion is observed at concentrations between 5×10^{-6} and 5×10^{-5}M, being indicative of a positive inotropic effect. At 10^{-4}M ouabain, arrhythmias are present.

5. Our data demonstrate the existence of one single class of cardiac glycoside receptors in cultured cardiac muscle cells from chicken embryos. In rat heart muscle cells, inhibition of the sodium pump, as well as positive inotropy, is coupled to occupation of the low affinity, high capacity cardiac glycoside receptor. In contrast, occupation of the high affinity, low capacity ouabain binding site of rat heart cells does not produce any measurable inhibition of sodium pump activity nor positive inotropy. Nature and function of this high affinity site remain to be elucidated.

Key words: cardiac glycosides, receptor, heart muscle cells, sodium pump, inotropy

Introduction

The discovery of different classes of ouabain binding sites in cardiac cell membranes from adult rats (4) has again stimulated the – still controversial – discussion of the mechanism of the positive inotropic action of cardiac glycosides (15). Subsequently, further experimental evidence has been presented, questioning sodium pump inhibition as the only mechanism of positive inotropic action of this drug: characterization of a high affinity receptor for cardiac glycosides in rat heart, coupled to positive inotropy, but not involved in sodium pump inhibition (4); bimodal inotropic response of the rat heart to cardiac glycosides (1, 6, 8, 11); existence of different forms of ($Na^+ + K^+$)-ATPase molecules (12, 13).

However, when discussing different forms of cardiac glycoside receptors and ($Na^+ + K^+$)-ATPase molecules in the heart, the parallel existence of cardiac muscle and non muscle cells has to be taken into account; the latter mainly consisting of fibroblasts and endothelial cells. Neither in cardiac cell membranes nor in cardiac muscle preparations, binding of cardiac glycosides to muscle cells can be distinguished from binding to cardiac non muscle cells. The demonstration of high and low affinity binding sites for ouabain in rat heart could therefore reflect different glycoside receptors in different classes of cardiac cells. For exclusion of this possibility, it is necessary to study separately cardiac glycoside binding to cardiac muscle as well as to cardiac non muscle cells.

From hearts of neonatal rats and chicken embryos, cultured cardiac muscle as well as non muscle cells can be obtained. We have used this established technique to characterize cardiac glycoside receptors in muscle and non muscle cells from both species (22, 23). The present paper concentrates on the question: does the intact rat heart muscle cell in culture indeed possess two different classes of cardiac glycoside receptors?

Materials and methods

Materials:

Chemicals were purchased from NEN Chemicals, D-6072 Dreieich, FRG ($^{22}Na^+$, carrier-free; $^{86}RbCl$, 0.9–4.6 mCi/mg; (^3H)-ouabain, 14–20 Ci/mmol); Biochrom, D-1000 Berlin, FRG (Collagenase "Worthington", 125–250 U/mg, CLS II; fetal calf serum; horse serum; CMRL 1415 ATM medium); Serva Biochemica, D-6900 Heidelberg, FRG (Trypsin 1:250, No 37290). All other chemicals were of analytical grade and purchased from Merck, D-6100 Darmstadt, FRG and from Boehringer-Mannheim, D-6800 Mannheim, FRG.

All *methods* used have been described in detail elsewhere (19, 20, 22, 23). In brief, the procedures are: *Cell culture techniques:* Muscle and non muscle cells from 50–200 hearts of 10–12 day-old chicken embryos and 1–3 day-old neonatal rats have been prepared under sterile conditions and separately cultured (19, 22, 23): disaggregation of the hearts by repeated incubation (10 min periods at 37°) in trypsin (0.12%)-collagenase (0.03%)-salt solution (Ca^{2+}, Mg^{2+} free); separate cultivation of muscle cells (seeding density about 10^5 cells/cm^2) and non muscle cells in 25 cm^2 plastic culture flasks (Nunclon plastics, DK-Roskilde, Denmark) at 37° after application of differential attachment technique, in growth medium (CMRL 1415 ATM, bicarbonate free, pH 7.40), supplemented with 10% fetal calf serum and 0.05 mg/ml gentamycin. The medium for cultivation of cardiac muscle cells was additionally supplemented with 10% horse serum. Experiments have been carried out with muscle cells after 2–3 days in culture, with non muscle cells after 1 subcultivation (splitting ratio 1:2, detachment of the cells by 0.05% trypsin + 0.02% EDTA in Ca^{2+}, Mg^{2+} free salt solution (Biochrom, Berlin)). At that time, muscle cells had formed a synchronously beating monolayer, non muscle cells were at confluency. The term "non muscle cells" refers to heart cells in culture, lacking sarcomeres, mainly consisting of fibroblasts and endothelial cells (19, 22).

Measurement of ($^{86}Rb^+ + K^+$)-influx, (^3H)-ouabain binding and cellular contents of Na^+ and K^+ in heart cells:

Standard measurements have been carried out at 37° with cells (0.2–2.0 mg protein/flask) in 25 cm^2 plastic flasks (incubation volume 4.1 ml) in serum-supplemented (2.5% fetal calf serum, 2.5% horse serum), Hepes buffered (20 mM, pH 7.40) CMRL 1415 ATM medium with lowered K^+concentration (0.75 mM). For measurement of the rate of active K^+ influx (20), cells have been incubated for 10 min with ($^{86}Rb^+$) in tracer amounts (2×10^6 cpm/flask); uptake linearly increased with time during this period; more than 90% of ($^{86}Rb^+ + K^+$)-influx could be inhibited by excess (10^{-3}M) of ouabain. Measurement of (^3H)-ouabain binding (about 3.5×10^6 cpm/flask) to the cells has been carried out in a similar manner (see also legend to fig. 1). Cellular K^+ contents have been measured by flame photometry, the exchangeable pool of intracellular Na^+ has been obtained by measurement of cellular $^{22}Na^+$ tracer under equilibrium conditions (20). For washing procedures, lysis of the cells, determination of cellular radioactivity and measurement of cellular protein according to the method of Lowry – using bovine serum albumin as standard – see (19, 20). The data presented in this report are means from closely correlating duplicates or triplicates. All experiments described have been carried out at least three times.

Results

Characterization of (^3H)-ouabain binding sites in cultured cardiac muscle cells from neonatal rats and chicken embryos

For comparison, binding experiments with cultured cardiac muscle cells have been carried out under identical conditions, both with cells from chicken embryos, as well as with cells from neonatal rats. In both cell types, (^{3}H)-ouabain binding is composed of specific and non specific binding. Three methods for measurement of non specific (^{3}H)-ouabain binding – which represents about 7% (chicken cells) and 17% (rat cells) of total binding at 10^{-7}M – have been applied, yielding identical results: binding to heat-denatured cells (60 min at 60°), binding in the presence of high K^+ (20 mM) or high ouabain (10^{-3}M) concentrations (22, 23). Specific (^{3}H)-ouabain binding to the cells is saturable within 30 min at 6×10^{-8}M, being stable for at least 6 hours. Concentration dependence of specific (^{3}H)-ouabain binding under equilibrium conditions is shown in the experiments of fig. 1 a:

in case of cardiac muscle cells from chicken embryos, saturation of binding is obtained at 10^{-6}M ouabain; in cardiac muscle cells from neonatal rats, however, specific binding increases up to 10^{-5}M ouabain, the highest concentration tested. Analysis of these binding data according to Scatchard (fig. 1 b) demonstrates a straight line in case of heart cells from chicken embryos, being indicative of a single class of ouabain binding sites. In case of heart cells from neonatal rats, on the other hand, a curved plot is obtained. As experimental evidence for negative cooperativity of binding is absent (see below), this finding indicates the presence of more than one class of ouabain binding sites in rat heart muscle cells: applying the program of Weidemann et al (18), binding data are compatible with the presence of two classes of ouabain binding sites: high affinity, low capacity sites, as well as low affinity, high capacity sites. Mean values for dissociation constants and binding capacities are given in table 1. Cardiac non muscle cells have fewer binding sites than cardiac muscle cells, but with similar binding affinities for ouabain: also one class of sites is present in chicken cells, but two classes in rat cells (22, 23).

The existence of one single class of binding sites in chicken heart cells, but of two classes in rat heart cells is further supported by different kinetics of ouabain binding process in these cells: in chicken heart cells, (^{3}H)-ouabain association follows second order, ouabain dissociation single first order reaction; the dissociation constant calculated from the rate constants being in good agreement with the one obtained from measurement of concentration-dependent ouabain binding under equilibrium conditions (22). In rat heart muscle cells, however, biphasic dissociation kinetics are present (table 1), the fast component being due to dissociation from the low affinity site ($t_{1/2} \leqq 12$ min at 37°). the slow component representing dissociation from the high affinity site ($t_{1/2} = 575$ min at 37°). High concentrations of ouabain (10^{-4}–10^{-3}M) do not alter kinetics of ouabain dissociation in rat heart muscle cells. Therefore, the existence of negative cooperativity of the binding sites can be excluded (3).

Further characterization of (^{3}H)-ouabain binding reveals a strong temperature dependency, as tested for binding to the sites in chicken heart cells and to the high affinity sites in rat heart muscle cells (table 1); binding to these sites is strongly suppressed by potassium ions, while ouabain dissociation from these sites is not altered by K^+ (22, 23).

Taking all experimental evidence together, our data demonstrate the existence of a single class of ouabain binding sites in cardiac muscle cells from chicken embryos, but of two classes of binding sites – about 10% high affinity sites and about 90% low affinity sites – in cardiac muscle cells from neonatal rats.

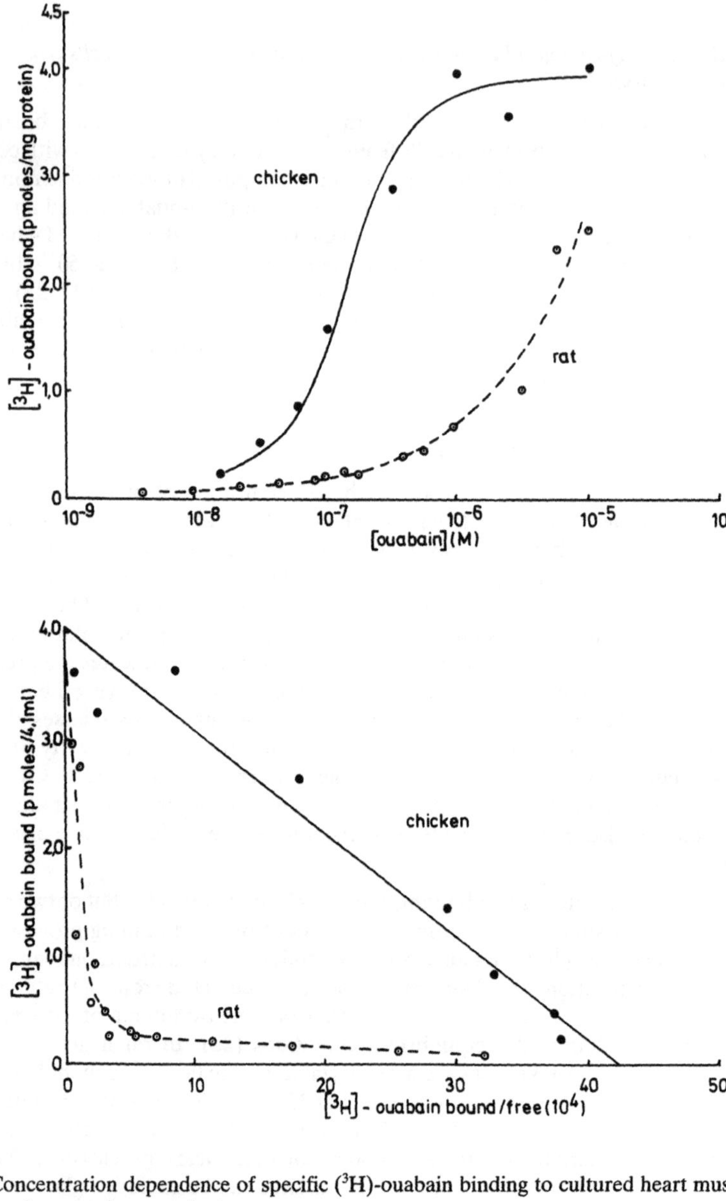

Fig. 1. Concentration dependence of specific (^{3}H)-ouabain binding to cultured heart muscle cells from chicken embryos and neonatal rats.

Fig. a. for measurement of (^{3}H)-ouabain binding, cells have been incubated for 4 hours at 37° in serum-supplemented, Hepes buffered CMRL medium ($[K^+]$ = 0.75 mM) in the presence of (^{3}H)-ouabain concentrations as indicated (see abscissa). For calculation of specific (^{3}H)-ouabain binding, non specific binding at 10^{-3}M ouabain (about 10% (chicken) and 20% (rat) of maximal counts bound) has been subtracted from total (^{3}H)-ouabain binding.

Fig. b. Scatchard plot analysis (16) of binding data presented in fig. a. Chicken cells: linear regression analysis yields the following results: B = 4.3 pmoles/mg protein; $K_D = 2.2 \times 10^{-7}$M; r = 0.98. Rat cells: analysis according to Weidemann et al (18) for two classes of binding sites yields the following values: B_1 = 0.2 pmoles/mg protein, $K_{D1} = 1.6 \times 10^{-8}$M; B_2 = 4.6 pmoles/mg protein, $K_{D2} = 8.9 \times 10^{-6}$M.

Table 1. Characterization of specific (^{3}H)-ouabain binding and of ouabain-induced inhibition of the sodium pump in cultured cardiac muscle cells from chicken embryos and neonatal rats. Values are given as mean from at least 3 experiments each. For further details see (22, 23).

	Cardiac muscle cells from Chicken embryos	Cardiac muscle cells from Neonatal rats	
Ouabain-induced inhibition of ($^{86}Rb^+ + K^+$)-influx (EC_{50},M)	5.8×10^{-7}	1.3×10^{-5}	
Ouabain-induced decrease in cellular K^+(EC_{50},M)	6.7×10^{-7}	1.9×10^{-5}	
Ouabain-induced increase in cellular Na^+(EC_{50},M)	7.4×10^{-7}	10^{-5}–10^{-4}	
		(^{3}H)-ouabain binding sites high affinity	low affinity
Dissociation constant K_D (M)	1.5×10^{-7}	3.2×10^{-8}	7×10^{-6}
Binding capacity			
pmoles/mg cell protein	2.6	0.2	2.6
sites/cell	8.6×10^5	8×10^4	10^6
Association rate constant k_{+1} ($M^{-1}s^{-1}$), 37°	3.2×10^4	$\sim1.5\times10^4$	
Dissociation rate constant k_{-1} (s^{-1}), 37°	4.5×10^{-3}	2×10^{-5}	$\geqq9\times10^{-4}$
Activation energy of			
association (kJ/mol), 9–36°	56	~70	
dissociation (kJ/mol), 9–36°	107	~90	
equilibrium binding (kJ/mol), 9–36°	–63		

Characterization of ouabain binding sites in heart muscle cells from chicken and rat as cardiac glycoside receptors

If ouabain binding sites – as characterized in the preceding section – represent cardiac glycoside receptors, then inhibition of the sodium pump and/or positive inotropic action should result from their occupation.

Sodium pump activity of cardiac muscle cells in culture has been monitored by measurement of ouabain-sensitive ($^{86}Rb^+ + K^+$)-influx (see methods). Concentration-dependent, progressive inhibition of ($^{86}Rb^+ + K^+$)-influx occurs at increasing ouabain concentrations in incubation medium, with EC_{50} values of 5.8×10^{-7}M (cardiac muscle cells from chicken embryos) and 1.3×10^{-5}M (cardiac muscle cells from neonatal rats), respectively. As consequence of sodium pump inhibition, cell-K^+ falls and cell-Na^+ rises (table 1). As can be seen from the experiments of fig. 2, occupation of the ouabain binding sites in chicken cells and occupation of the low affinity binding sites in rat cells are correlated with inhibition of the sodium pump. In contrast, binding of ouabain to the high affinity sites in rat cells does not inhibit ($^{86}Rb^+ + K^+$)-influx.

Increase in amplitude and velocity of cell wall motion represents the equivalent of positive inotropic action in beating cardiac muscle cells in culture (9, 17). In case of cultured cardiac muscle cells from chicken embryos, a concentration-dependent increase in amplitude of cell wall motion is observed between 10^{-7} and 10^{-6}M ouabain (2). The dissociation constant (1.5×10^{-7}M) for specific (^{3}H)-ouabain binding to these cells is within the same concentration range (figs. 1, 2, table 1), demonstrating close coupling of ouabain binding to its binding sites and positive inotropic action.

For beating heart muscle cells from neonatal rats, the concentration-dependent increase in velocity of cell wall motion by ouabain is shown in fig. 3: while 5×10^{-7} and 10^{-6}M ouabain are without any influence, clear-cut increases are shown at 5×10^{-6}-5×10^{-5}M ouabain. A further increase in ouabain concentration (10^{-4}M) leads to arrhythmias. The ouabain effect on contractility is readily reversible: it can be washed out within 5 min (23).

Discussion

High and low affinity ouabain binding sites were first demonstrated in cardiac cell membranes from adult rats (4, 5). This finding can now be extended to the intact rat heart muscle cell: with all experiments carried out under identical conditions, one single class of

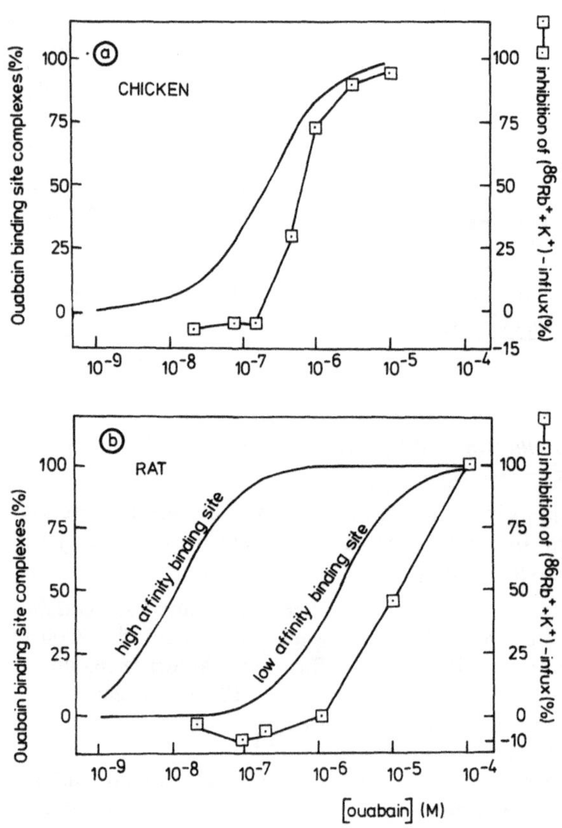

Fig. 2. Effect of (^{3}H)-ouabain binding to its binding sites on ouabain-sensitive ($^{86}Rb^+ + K^+$)-influx rate in cultured cardiac muscle cells from chicken embryos and neonatal rats. Concentration-dependent, specific (^{3}H)-ouabain binding has been carried out and analysed according to Scatchard as described in the experiments of fig. 1. Based on the measured K_D-values, application of law of mass action allows construction of the curves for binding site occupancy (–). Chicken cells: $K_D = 2.0 \times 10^{-7}$M; rat cells: K_{D1} (high affinity site) $= 1.1 \times 10^{-8}$M, K_{D2} (low affinity site) $= 1.7 \times 10^{-6}$M. ($^{86}Rb^+ + K^+$)-influx rates have been obtained by incubation of the cells for 5 min with ($^{86}Rb^+$), after a preincubation period of 4 hours at the appropriate ouabain concentration; $[K^+] = 0.75$ mM. From the amount of ($^{86}Rb^+ + K^+$) taken up, initial transport rates for ($^{86}Rb^+ + K^+$) have been calculated (20).

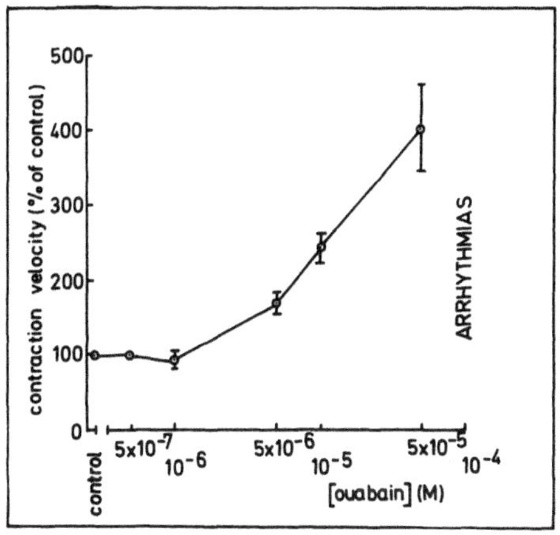

Fig. 3. Effect of ouabain on velocity of cell wall motion in rat heart muscle cells in culture. Beating of electrically driven (pacing rate 100/min; 100 V; pulse duration 10 msec) rat heart muscle cells – cultured on glass coverslips – has been monitored under a phase contrast microscope, using an electro-optical monitoring system ((19); 37°; superfusion of the cells (4 ml/min) with serum-free, Hepes buffered incubation medium (CMRL 1415 with modified Ca^{2+} (0.3 mM) and K^+ (1.5 mM) concentrations)). During course of observation, velocity of cell wall motion has been registered every 30 sec. After a control period of 5 min, ouabain at different concentrations has been added to the perfusion medium. After reaching a new steady state level of velocity of cell wall motion (10 min), ouabain has been washed out by superfusion of the cells with ouabain-free medium; the ouabain effect being readily reversible within 5 min. Velocity of cell wall motion is given as mean ± SEM (n = 3–10), as % of control. Only one ouabain concentration has been tested with each single cell.

ouabain binding sites has been found in cultured cardiac muscle cells from chicken embryos, but two classes of ouabain binding sites are present in rat heart muscle cells. This experimental evidence comes from both: measurement of (^{3}H)-ouabain binding under equilibrium conditions, as well as kinetic studies of (^{3}H)-ouabain binding processes. Results obtained with cardiac cell membranes – prepared from the same tissues as cultured heart cells – further support the existence of different classes of ouabain binding sites in hearts from neonatal rats (22, 23).

In presenting our results, it should be emphasized that work from other laboratories has shown the existence of a single class of saturable high affinity ouabain binding sites (14), as well as the presence of saturable high affinity and non saturable low affinity ouabain binding sites in cultured heart cells from neonatal rats (7); in cardiocytes from adult rats, also a high affinity binding site for ouabain has been described (1). In contrast to our results, high and low affinity binding sites for cardiac glycosides have been also found to occur in cultured cardiac muscle cells from chicken embryos (10); the reason for these contradictory results remains to be clarified.

The single class of ouabain binding sites (about 10^6 sites/cell) – as found under our experimental conditions – in cardiac muscle cells from chicken embryos (fig. 1) fulfills the criteria of a cardiac glycoside receptor: binding of ouabain to these sites results in a positive inotropic effect (2), as well as in inhibition of the sodium pump (fig. 2a). Though no linear coupling of receptor occupancy and sodium pump inhibition exists in chicken cardiac muscle cells (fig. 2a; for discussion see ref. 21, 22), a linear correlation has been found in cardiac non muscle cells from this species (21, 22).

In case of cultured cardiac muscle cells from neonatal rats, both pharmacological actions of cardiac glycosides can be attributed to occupation of the low affinity, high capacity ouabain binding site (10^6 sites/cell): inhibition of the sodium pump (fig. 2b), as well as positive inotropic action (fig. 3).

The role of the high affinity, low capacity site of rat heart cells (8×10^4 sites/cell), on the other hand, remains to be elucidated: an involvement of this site in sodium pump inhibition can be clearly ruled out, as has been shown for cultured cells (fig. 2b, (23)), as well as for heart tissue of adult rats (4). It remains to be confirmed, whether this site indeed represents part of the (Na^+ + K^+)-ATPase molecule (12, 13). No experimental evidence exists at present, demonstrating that occupation of this high affinity site is coupled to positive inotropy in these cells, though this coupling has been clearly shown to occur in ventricular strips from adult rats (1, 4, 11). The reason for this discrepancy is unknown: it may result from methodological limitations of the monitoring system used to measure small increases in amplitude and velocity of cell wall motion (23); coupling of the high affinity receptor with the positive inotropic event may be development-dependent and not be fully established in the cardiocytes of neonatal rats; coupling may be destroyed by the trypsin-collagenase treatment of the heart and may not be fully repaired or renewed during the cell culture period.

At present, three methodological approaches indicate the presence of high and low affinity cardiac glycoside receptors in rat heart: work with cardiac cell membranes, with cardiac muscle preparations and with beating heart muscle cells in culture. Based on the results obtained with cultured rat heart cells, it can be ruled out that the different types of cardiac glycoside receptors only represent receptors of different cell types (e.g. muscle and non muscle cells) of the rat heart.

The expert technical assistance of B. Walther is gratefully acknowledged. This work was supported by the Wilhelm-Sander-Stiftung (78.014.3) and by Deutsche Forschungsgemeinschaft (Er 65/4–3).

References

1. Adams RJ, Schwartz A, Grupp G, Grupp I, Lee SW, Wallick ET (1982) High-affinity ouabain binding site and low-dose positive inotropic effect in rat myocardium. Nature 296:167–169
2. Biedert St, Barry WH, Smith TW (1979) Inotropic effects and changes in sodium and calcium contents associated with inhibition of monovalent cation active transport by ouabain in cultured myocardial cells. J Gen Physiol 74:479–494
3. De Meyts P, Roth J, Neville DM, Gavin JR, Lesniak MA (1973) Insulin interactions with its receptors: experimental evidence for negative cooperativity. Biochem Biophys Res Commun 55:154–161
4. Erdmann E, Philipp G, Scholz H (1980) Cardiac glycoside receptor, (Na^+ +K^+)-ATPase activity and force of contraction in rat heart. Biochem Pharmacol 29:3219–3229
5. Erdmann E (1981) Influence of cardiac glycosides on their receptor. In "Handbook of experimental pharmacology", Vol 56/I cardiac glycosides (ed. Greeff K), Springer Verlag Berlin, 337–380
6. Finet M, Noel F, Godfraind T (1982) Inotropic effect and binding sites of ouabain to rat heart. Arch int Pharmacodyn 256:168–170
7. Friedman I, Schwalb H, Hallaq H, Pinson A, Heller M (1980) Interaction of cardiac glycosides with cultured cardiac cells. II. Biochemical and electron microscopic studies on the effects of ouabain on muscle and non muscle cells. Biochim Biophys Acta 598:272–284
8. Grupp IL, Grupp G, Schwartz A (1981) Digitalis receptor desensitization in rat ventricle: ouabain produces two inotropic effects. Life Sciences 29:2789–2794

9. Kaufmann R, Tritthart H, Rodenroth S, Rost B (1969) Das mechanische und elektrische Verhalten isolierter embryonaler Herzmuskelzellen in Zellkulturen. Pflügers Arch 311:25–49
10. Kazazoglou T, Renaud JF, Rossi B, Lazdunski M (1983) Two classes of ouabain receptors in chick ventricular cardiac cells and their relation to (Na^+, K^+)-ATPase inhibition, intracellular Na^+ accumulation, Ca^{2+} influx, and cardiotonic effect. J Biol Chem 258:12163–12170
11. Koomen JM, van Gilst WH, Zimmerman ANE, van Nordwijk J (1982) A concentration-dependent biphasic positive inotropic action of ouabain on isolated hearts of rat and guinea pig. Arch int Pharmacodyn 255:212–219
12. Mansier P, Lelievre LG (1982) Ca^{2+}-free perfusion of rat heart reveals a (Na^+ +K^+)-ATPase form highly sensitive to ouabain. Nature 300, 535–537
13. Mansier P, Cassidy PS, Charlemagne D, Preteseille M, Lelievre LG (1983) Three Na^+, K^+-ATPase forms in rat heart as revealed by K^+/ouabain antagonism. FEBS Letters 153:357–360
14. McCall D (1979) Cation exchange and glycoside binding in cultured rat heart cells. Am J Physiol 236:C87–C95
15. Noble D (1980) Mechanism of action of therapeutic levels of cardiac glycosides. Cardiovascular Res 14:495–514
16. Scatchard G (1949) The attractions of proteins for small molecules and ions. Ann NY Acad Sci 51:660–672
17. Schanne OF, Bkaily G (1981) Explanted cardiac cells: a model to study drug actions? Can J Physiol Pharmacol 59:443–467
18. Weidemann MJ, Erdelt H, Klingenberg M (1970) Adenine nucleotide translocation of mitochondria. Identification of carrier sites. Eur J Biochem 16:313–335
19. Werdan K, Bauriedel G, Bozsik M, Krawietz W, Erdmann E (1980) Effects of vanadate in cultured rat heart muscle cells. Vanadate transport, intracellular binding and vanadate-induced changes in beating and in active cation flux. Biochim Biophys Acta 597:364–383
20. Werdan K, Bauriedel G, Fischer B, Krawietz W, Erdmann, Schmitz W, Scholz H (1982) Stimulatory (insulin-mimetic) and inhibitory (ouabain-like) action of vanadate on potassium uptake and cellular sodium and potassium in heart cells in culture. Biochim Biophys Acta 687:79–93
21. Werdan K, Zwißler B, Wagenknecht B, Krawietz W, Erdmann E (1983) Quantitative correlation of cardiac glycoside binding to its receptor and inhibition of the sodium pump in chicken heart cells in culture. Biochem Pharmacol 32:757–760
22. Werdan K, Wagenknecht B, Zwißler B, Brown L, Krawietz W, Erdmann E (1984) Cardiac glycoside receptors in cultured heart cells: I. Characterization of one single class of high affinity receptors in heart muscle cells from chick embryos. Biochem Pharmacol, 33:55–70
23. Werdan K, Wagenknecht B, Zwißler B, Brown L, Krawietz W, Erdmann E Cardiac glycoside receptors in cultured heart cells. II. Characterization of a high affinity and a low affinity binding site in heart muscle cells from neonatal rats. Biochem Pharmacol, in press

Authors' address:

Dr. Karl Werdan, Medizinische Klinik I, Klinikum Großhadern, Marchioninisstr. 15, D-8000 München 70 (FRG)

Binding sites for ouabain in human and rat erythrocytes and in rat heart cells

M. Heller

Laboratory for Myocardial Research, Institute of Biochemistry, Hebrew University – Hadassah Medical School, Jerusalem (Israel)

Summary

The presence and properties of two classes of binding sites for digitalis in erythrocytes and in heart cells are reviewed. Methods to distinguish between these two binding sites are summarized for intact cells and for their membranes. Our biochemical data do not suggest a physiological role for each class of sites.

The membrane sites were modified by varying (a) the content of cholesterol or (b) the distribution of fatty acids leading to changes in the microviscosity thus affecting the degree of binding of ouabain to the two classes of sites. Oxidation of ouabain with periodate forms a di-aldehyde which could bind via Schiff base to the digitalis sites but could also attach covalently to these sites. The role of the sugar moiety in the process of ouabain binding becomes of increasing importance.

A mild, controlled periodate oxidation of ouabain, especially in presence of phosphate cleaves only the bond between C-2 and C-3 of the rhamnose without affecting the steroid moiety. The periodate oxidation provided additional information for assigning a distorted chair conformation or a transient boat conformation for rhamnose in ouabain. It was also established by ^{1}H NMR spectroscopy that this chair conformation is a $^1C_4$ pyranose ring.

Key words: Cardiomyocytes, erythrocytes, membrane lipids, receptors, ouabain

Introduction

The existence of more than one class of binding sites for digitalis in hearts from guinea pigs, dogs, rats or humans, has been suggested by a number of investigators (1, 2, 5, 6, 8, 9, 14, 20). Some of the proposals have indicated the presence of (Na^+ + K^+)-ATPase isoenzymes as a plausible explanation, and indeed such iso-forms were described in rat brain, adipocytes and brine shrimps with different affinities for cardiac glycosides (15, 16, 18). On the other hand, it was also claimed that in spite of the existence of isoenzymes not all of them necessarily bear any relation to digitalis binding sites or to regulation of transport functions.

In our earlier studies on human and rat erythrocytes, as well as post-natal rat cultured heart cells, we have also reached the conclusion that two classes of binding sites for ouabain exist. The hydrophilic ouabain was chosen as a tool for specific binding because of its relatively low lipid solubility, reduced penetration into intracellular spaces and minimal non-specific binding. This also ruled out the possibility to assign internal membraneous location for one of the binding classes at least in intact cells.

Methods

Preparation of human or rat erythrocytes, post-natal rat cardiac muscle or non-muscle cells, their respective membranes and the conditions for measuring binding of ^{3}H-ouabain, were previously described (7, 11, 12, 19).

The details for the modifications of membrane compositions were published earlier (3, 13). The conditions for oxidation of ouabain by $NaIO_4$ were either those of Butler and Smith (17) or alternatively together with the determination of the conformation of rhamnose and ouabain, are still unpublished results (10).

Results and discussion

A. Binding of ouabain to erythrocytes and heart cells

The two classes of sites were distinguished on the basis of equilibrium binding of the drug in absence or presence of K^+ (about 10 mM). The sites are thus referred to as "potassium sensitive" and "potassium insensitive". K^+ affected the binding only at concentrations of ouabain below 1 μM (7, 11). The duration of exposure in heart cells was minimal (less than 30 min.), to avoid cell damage due to absence of K^+. The $[K^+]_{1/2}$ for these cells was 1.5 mM, a value far below the normal range of 3.5–5 mM at which concentration ouabain is expected to bind to the K^+– insensitive sites (1, 19).

Equilibrium binding of ouabain showed saturability to the potassium insensitive sites at about 1 μM with high affinity, whereas the low affinity sites required much higher concentration of ouabain (7, 11).

Cardiac tissue is composed of muscle and non-muscle cells. In both types of cells the two classes of sites were detected, and the K_D values and number of total sites per cell at the high affinity range of ouabain concentration were determined. In these cells it was also observed that the number of ouabain molecules bound per muscle cell declines as the culture ages. An overgrowth of non-muscle cells as an explanation was ruled out. A process of "receptor-ageing" was proposed to explain this decrease in the number of the high affinity sites, since the experiment was done with 7.5 nM ouabain. This information may be related to the decrease in the sensitivity of rats toward the pharmacological action of ouabain as the newborn rat matures (7, 12, 19).

B. Binding of ouabain to membranes

1. Erythrocytes

The existence of two classes of binding sites was demonstrated in membrane vesicles obtained from human or rat erythrocytes. The distinction in these preparations between the sites is based on "activation" of the receptors, achieved by exposing them to $Na^+ + Mg^{2+} +$ ATP, or to $Mg^{2+} + P_i$. The receptors in their phosphorylated or otherwise forms apparently acquire a favorable conformation which allows high affinity binding of cardiac glycosides. Another conformation which may or may not be phosphorylated exists with a low affinity for forming a complex with ouabain. The sites with high affinity are obtained by subtraction from the total binding obtained in the presence of $Mg^{2+} + P_i$ of the binding obtained in the absence of $Mg^{2+} + P_i$ which represents the low affinity sites. These two sites are referred to as *type I* and *type II* for the low and high affinity sites respectively.

Further distinction between the sites in human erythrocytes was made, based on the following:

(a) Only type II sites (high affinity) are sensitive to cations in the order $K^+ > Na^+ > Cs^+$ with I_{50} of 1, 7.5 and 22 mM, respectively.
(b) Storage of membranes at –20 °C for 56 days affected type I (low affinity) sites only but subsequent storage caused rapid deterioration of both types of sites with a $[t]_{1/2}$ of about 10 days.

(c) Extraction of human erythrocyte membranes with dry ether removed cholesterol and phospholipids, caused partial damage to type I (low affinity) sites (about 40%) and complete loss of type II (high affinity) binding capacity. Microsomal lipids, devoid of cholesterol, restored type I (low affinity) sites completely and type II (high affinity) sites to about 40% of maximal at 0.1 mg and 0.5 mg phospholipid per mg membrane protein, respectively.

(d) Possible interconversion between the two types of sites was excluded by the following experiments: Membranes exposed to 42 nM ^3H ouabain alone yielded equilibrium binding values corresponding to type I sites only. If first incubated with ouabain then Mg^{2+} + P_i added and incubation continued for a total fixed period both classes of sites became labelled in an additive manner. If phosphorylated first with Mg^{2+} + P_i in the absence of ouabain and then incubated with the drug for the same total fixed period, only type II sites became labelled (11).

The fixation of the proper conformation of type II (high affinity) sites requires the presence and/or binding of ouabain.

Transformation of one class of sites to the other could not be demonstrated. At lower concentrations of ouabain, e.g. below 1 μM, type II sites predominate whereas at higher concentrations, above 1 μM, type I sites prevail. Rat erythrocyte membranes displayed primarily sites of type I even at the lower range of ouabain concentrations (11, 12).

C. Modifications

1. Heart cells

The role of lipids in binding of ouabain has been mentioned above. Consequently an approach was adopted in which the content of the sarcolemmal cholesterol was modified by supplementing the medium with cholesterol, increasing the amount of cholesterol in the sarcolemma by 20–30% with minimal damage to the cells (12). Alternatively, the sarcolemmal fatty acid composition was shifted either toward a more saturated one or more unsaturated one by growing the cells in the presence of stearic acid $C_{18:0}$ or erucic acid $C_{22:1}$ respectively. Relaxation time (τ_0) measurements of a spin label probe reflected the changes in the microviscosity of these sarcolemma: stearic acid (as well as cholesterol) caused increases in viscosity, membranes were less fluid, whereas erucic acid – the opposite, membranes were less viscous, more fluid. Fatty acid analysis of sarcolemmal lipids supported these data (3, 13).

The decrease in sarcolemmal fluidity by supplementation with cholesterol or the increase of the fluidity due to shift in unsaturation was also reflected in the binding of ouabain to the two classes of sites using 7.5 nM ouabain as follows (cf. Table I):

(a) "Potassium insensitive" sites (= type I receptors) – cholesterol increased binding capacity by 15 times, erucic acid – none.

(b) "Potassium sensitive" sites (= type II receptors) – cholesterol had no effect, erucic acid caused 50% reduction in binding.

It may be suggested that the low affinity sites (i.e. type I) are squeezed out by the solidification of the membrane with excess cholesterol but are unaffected by the liquification of the membranes. On the contrary, the high-affinity sites (type II) do not respond to the solidification but sink deeper into the membrane when they become more fluid.

2. Erythrocytes

With erythrocytes the following techniques were employed in an attempt to characterize, differentially, the two classes of binding sites:

(a) Enrichment or depletion of intact human cells or their membranes with respect to

Table 1. Alteration of lipid content and ouabain binding by cultured cardiac cells

μg cholesterol / plate	or	μmole erucic acid / plate	binding site	10^{-14}moles ouabain/mg protein	
				cholesterol	erucic acid
49		0	"K^+	0.15	2.90
83		1	insensitive"	1.80	2.97
49		0	"K^+	6.25	2.00
83		1	sensitive"	6.30	1.07

Plates containing approximately 10^6 myocytes in Tyrode solution ± 2.68 mM K^+ were incubated with 7.5 nM ^3H-ouabain. The amounts of either cholesterol or erucic acid affecting the binding of ouabain are shown.

cholesterol, or alternatively, partial replacement with cholestenone (3 – oxidized cholesterol). The parameters measured included the activities of the Na^+, K^+-ATPase and K^+-phosphatase as well as binding of ouabain. Although useful information was obtained it did not provide a clearer picture (12).

(b) Formation of sealed, right side out or inside out membrane vesicles at a high degreee of purity was very encouraging in providing preliminary results at this stage. This approach requires further elaboration for complete exploitation.

(c) Replacement of ouabain by periodate-oxidized ouabain as a probe. This approach seems to provide interesting data, some of which is given below as well as an auxilliary means for studying the structure and conformation of ouabain (12).

Oxidation of ouabain with $NaIO_4$ has been applied in the past by a number of groups for various purposes, mainly for the formation of a more functional entity such as aldehyde, to form a Schiff base with free amino groups. The published procedures describe the use of a large excess of periodate for the oxidation (10, 17).

It was anticipated that the more reactive di-aldehyde group in the oxidized rhamnose moiety of ouabain, after saturating the binding sites, will form an aldimide (Schiff base) with free NH_2 groups at the "sugar site" of the receptor or at a close vicinity to it. The Schiff base may be further stabilized by reduction with $NaBH_4$ (10).

The binding of oxidized ouabain to the two classes of sites was compared to that of ouabain, at 4 nM each, with and without the step of $NaBH_4$ reduction. Extraction of the complexes with methanol or perchloric acid was applied to confirm the covalent binding of the oxidized ouabain to both classes of the binding sites. At this stage the data is insufficient to provide diagnostic means for clear differentiation of the two sites (12).

D. Conformation of rhamnose in ouabain

The experiments with oxidized ouabain have led us to reconsider the role of the sugar moiety in the process of binding. It has been shown that when (Mg^{2+} + P_i) was employed for the binding of glycosides, the dissociation rate constant is dependent upon the sugar moiety. The steroid portion binds to the receptors first, induces a conformation change which leads to an activation of the sugar binding sites (22).

In general, much less attention has been paid to the analysis of the binding of the sugar moiety although it seems now that more publications deal with this aspect.

The contribution of the sugar moiety to the effectiveness and stability of complex formation between the receptor and the glycoside has shown that L-rhamnosides, e.g. ouabain, tend to

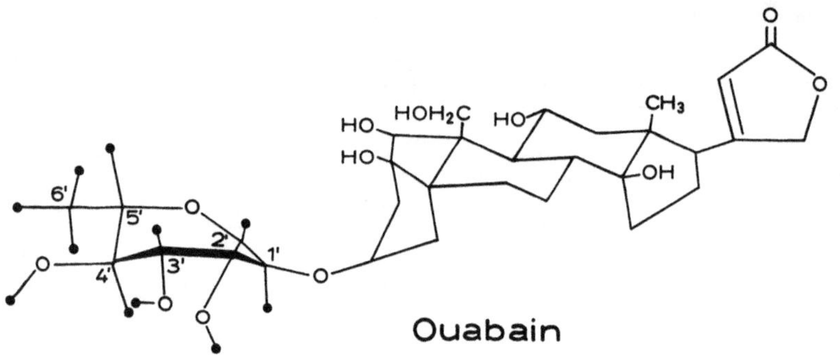

Fig. 1. Proposal of the proper conformation of ouabain based on ^{1}H-NMR studies of the intact and $NaIO_4$ oxidized cardiac glycoside (21).

form the most stable complexes. Based on Molecular Rotation data presented by Klyne in 1950, a structure of rhamnose in ouabain was a $^{4}C_{1}$ chair conformation and an axially oriented hydroxyl group attached to C-3 of rhamnose (22). Based on this structure, the crucial hydroxyl group participating in the binding of the rhamnose is the C-3-OH which is expected to form a double hydrogen bond with a proton donor group (X) and a proton acceptor group (Y) at the membrane binding site (22). This forms a stable complex but only when the hydroxyl is axially oriented. Equatorially oriented hydroxyl forms, according to this mechanism, only a single hydrogen bond with the acceptor Y group, hence lower stability. This proposal was based on studies with glycosides having the proper oriented C-3-OH group, as well as C-3 methoxy group to support this thesis. Recently this mechanism was challenged in a similar study in which the cardiotonic activity of different glycosides was examined (4). Although a different conformational assignment for the bound rhamnose was shown, i.e. a $^{1}C_{4}$ chair of the pyranose ring with the hydroxyls attached to C-2, C-4 and methyl of C-5 are equatorially oriented and not axial as was previously suggested, the orientation of the C-3-OH even in this new conformation remained axial. This study has shown that methoxy group at C-3 has very little effect on the drug's potency and reached the conclusion that the free rotation about the glycosidic linkage allows the aquisition of any desired conformation – an induced fit concept (4).

We have recently confirmed the conformation of $^{1}C_{4}$ chair of the rhamnoside pyranose ring in ouabain using ^{1}H NMR spectroscopy (21). A proper assignment of each proton in the rhamnose as well as certain protons of the steroid moiety was made. Support for the proposed structure was obtained from a periodate oxidized molecule of ouabain which was done under much milder conditions than that published earlier, namely using only one equivalent of $NaIO_4$ and obligatory presence of two equivalents of KH_2PO_4 for no longer than 60 min at room temperature. Under these circumstances, only the bond between C-2 and C-3 of the rhamnose was cleaved. Under previously published procedures, the oxidation went beyond the stage of aldehyde and affected also the steroid nucleus such as the vinylic hydrogen, resulting in low yields of the desired product and adding damaged, probably pharmacologically inactive glycoside. The entire information gathered from these studies supported a $^{1}C_{4}$ chair or rather a distorted chair, which may also have properties of a transient boat conformation. (Fig. 1).

With these data, it may be possible to proceed in the attempts to approach the problems associated with the interaction of cardiac glycosides with their respective binding sites.

Acknowledgements:

The author wishes to thank all the collaborators who participated in these studies. The studies described were supported in part by grants obtained from the Chief Scientists, Ministries of Health and of Commerce and Industry; Schönbrunn Foundation.

References

1. Adams RJ, Schwartz A, Grupp G, Grupp I, Lee SW, Wallick ET, Powell T, Twist VW, Gathiram P (1982) High-affinity ouabain binding site and low-dose positive inotropic effect in rat myocardium. Nature 296:167–168
2. Barry WH, Biedert S, Miura DS, Smith TW (1981) Changes in cellular Na^+, K^+, and Ca^{++} contents, monovalent cation transport rate, and contractile state during washout of cardiac glycosides from cultured chick heart cells. Circ Res 49:141–149
3. Benenson A, Heller M, Pinson A, Mersel M (1982) Advances in studies on heart metabolism, ed Caldarera CM and Harris P, pp 49–56, Proteolipid and lipid moieties in Sarcolemma
4. Brown L, Thomas R (1983) Comparison of the inotropic potencies of some synthetic and naturally occurring cardiac glycosides using isolated left atrium of guinea pig. Arzneim Forsch 33:814–817
5. Erdmann E, Philipp G, Scholz H (1980) Cardiac glycoside receptor, ($Na^+ + K^+$)-ATPase activity and force of contraction in rat heart. Biochem Pharmacol 29:3219–3229
6. Erdmann E, Brown L, Krawietz W, Werdan K (1983) Quantitative evaluation of ^{3}H-ouabain binding to contracting heart muscle, positive inotropy, Na,K-ATPase inhibition, and $^{86}Rb^+$ uptake in several species. In: Hoffmann JF, Forbush B (eds) Current Topics in Membranes and Transport, Vol 19, Structure, mechanism and function of Na/K pump. Academic Press, New York, p 891–895
7. Friedman I, Schwalb H, Hallaq H, Pinson A, Heller M (1980) Interactions of cardiac glycosides with cultured cardiac cells. Biochim Biophys Acta 598:272–284
8. Godfraind T (1981) In: Greeff K (ed) Handbook of Experimental Pharmacology, Vol 56/1 p 381
9. Grupp IL, Grupp G, Schwartz A (1981) Digitalis receptor desensitization in rat ventricle: Ouabain produces two inotropic effects. Life Sci 29:2789–2794
10. Hegyvary C (1975) Covalent labeling of the digitalis-binding component of plasma membranes. Mol Pharmacol 11:588–594
11. Heller M, Beck S (1978) Interactions of cardiac glycosides with cells and membranes. Biochim Biophys Acta 514:332–347
12. Heller M, Beck S, Friedman I, Hallaq H, Mersel M, Pinson A, Schwalb H, Smith E, Yehiel E (1979) Intl Symp of Intl Soc Heart Research, pp 97–110, Digitalis and the plasma membrane
13. Mersel M, Amar A, Benenson A, Heller M, Hallaq H, Padieu P, Pinson A (1982) Advances in studies on heart metabolism, ed Caldarera CM and Harris P, pp 89–93, Sarcolemma fluidity
14. Noble D (1980) Mechanism of action of therapeutic levels of cardiac glycosides. Cardiovasc Res 14:495–514
15. Peterson GL, Churchill L, Fisher JA, Hokin LE (1982) Structure and biosynthesis of (Na,K)-ATPase in developing brine shrimp Nauplii. Ann NY Acad Sci 402:185–191
16. Resh MD, Nemenoff RA, Guidotti G (1980) Insulin stimulation of (Na,K)-adenosine triphosphatase-dependent $^{86}Rb^+$ uptake in rat adipocytes. J Biol Chem 255:10938–10945
17. Smith TW, Butler VP Jr, Haber E (1970) Characterization of antibodies of high affinity and specificity for the digitalis glycoside digoxin. Biochemistry 9:331–337
18. Sweadner KJ (1979) Two molecular forms of ($Na^+ + K^+$)-stimulated ATPase in brain. J Biol Chem 254:6060–6067
19. Schwalb H, Dickstein Y, Heller M (1982) Interactions of cardiac glycosides with cardiac cells. Biochim Biophys Acta 689:241–248
20. Schwartz A, Whitmer K, Grupp G, Grupp I, Adams RJ, Lee SW (1983) Mechanism of action of digitalis: Is the Na,K-ATPase the pharmacological receptor? Ann. NY Acad Sci 402:253–259
21. Yanuka Y, Hallaq H, Heller M (1984) Submitted to Biochem Biophys Res Comm
22. Yoda A (1973) Structure-acitivity relationships of cardiotonic steroids for the inhibition of sodium- and potassium-dependent adenosine triphosphatase. Mol Pharmacol 9:51–60

Author's address:

Prof. Dr. Michael Heller, Laboratory for Myocardial Research, Institute of Biochemistry-Hebrew Univ.-Hadassah Med. School, P.O.B. 1172, Jerusalem (Israel) 91010

Two binding sites for ouabain in cardiac cell membranes

L.Brown and E. Erdmann

Medizinische Klinik I der Universität, Klinikum Grosshadern, München (FRG)

Summary

Cardiac glycoside receptors were defined by simultaneous measurement of ^{3}H-ouabain binding and its effects on cardiac cell membranes, contracting cardiac muscle and cultured cardiac cells. These measurements show that:

1. Rat and guinea pig cardiac cell membranes have two specific ouabain binding sites.

2. In both species, ouabain binding to the high affinity site on cell membranes correlates with the positive inotropic effect in contracting cardiac muscle. Inhibition of (Na^{+} + K^{+})-ATPase activity corresponds to binding to the low affinity site. This questions the hypothesis that (Na^{+} + K^{+})-ATPase inhibition is necessary for ouabain-induced positive inotropy.

3. K^{+} may induce an heterogeneity in the ouabain binding sites of the digitalis-sensitive cat and human heart.

*Key words:*ouabain, cardiac cell membranes, inotropy, (Na^{+} + K^{+})-ATPase activity

Introduction

A widely accepted hypothesis is that cardiac glycosides exert their pharmacological effects after binding to a specific receptor which is part of the (Na^{+} + K^{+})-ATPase, the enzyme responsible for active Na^{+} and K^{+} transport (1). The relationship between binding and pharmacological effects can be seen when ^{3}H-ouabain binding, force of contraction and $^{42}K^{+}$- or $^{86}Rb^{+}$-uptake (as measures of (Na^{+} + K^{+})-ATPase activity in contracting heart muscle and cultured cardiac cells) are measured simultaneously (2–4). Since the cardiac glycoside receptor is part of the cell membrane, this receptor can be further defined by measurement of ouabain binding and its consequences in partially purified cell membranes. To do this, cell membranes enriched in (Na^{+} + K^{+})-ATPase have been incubated under a variety of conditions, including conditions which more closely approximate experiments with contracting cardiac muscle.

Materials and methods

Materials:

^{3}H-Ouabain (specific activity 18 Ci/mmol, lot no. 1357–171) was purchased from New England Nuclear, Dreieich, Germany. All other chemicals were of analytical grade and were obtained from Boehringer Mannheim, Mannheim, Germany or E. Merck, Darmstadt, Germany.

Preparation of (Na^{+} + K^{+})-ATPase-containing cell membranes from beef, cat, human, guinea pig and neonatal rat hearts:

The partial purification procedure using sodium deoxycholate and sodium iodide extractions has been previously described (2, 3). The deoxycholate-treated enzyme from human and neonatal rat hearts homogenized in 1 mM EDTA, pH 7.25, was used without further purification. The (Na^{+} + K^{+})-ATPase activity, determined by the coupled optical assay (5), was between 0.1 and 0.3 μmole ATP hydrolyzed /

min / mg protein at 37 ° for the sodium iodide-treated enzyme suspensions and 0.02–0.15 µmole ATP hydrolyzed / min / mg protein at 37 ° for the sodium deoxycholate-treated enzyme suspensions. Protein was determined by the method of Lowry et al (6), using bovine serum albumin as standard. About 90–95 % of the total (N^+ + K^+)-ATPase activity of the NaI-treated cell membranes was inhibited by 1 × 10^{-3}M ouabain; for the deoxycholate-treated cell membranes, 1 × 10^{-3}M ouabain inhibited the activity by 70–85 %.

^{3}H-Ouabain binding and inhibition of (Na^+ + K^+)-ATPase activity:

The procedures used for these experiments have been described elsewhere (2,3). The following incubation media with about 2 – 8 × 10^{-9}M ^{3}H-ouabain were used: 1. 3 mM $MgCl_2$, 3 mM imidazole/PO_4 in 50 mM imidazole/HCl, pH 7.25; 2. 150 mM NaCl, 3 mM ATP, 3 mM $MgCl_2$ in 50 mM imidazole/HCl, pH 7.25; 3. 3 mM ATP in Tyrode solution, pH 7.4. The total volume for all binding assays was 2 ml. Incubation time was 1h (neonatal rat heart), 2h (guinea pig heart) or 3h (cat, human and beef heart cell membranes).

Results

Ouabain binding to cardiac cell membranes from cat, human and guinea pig and ouabain inhibition of (Na^+ + K^+)-ATPase have been measured. In the guinea pig cardiac cell membranes, in contrast to cat and human cell membranes, ouabain binding occurred without a corresponding inhibition of (Na^+ + K^+)-ATPase activity (3). Ouabain binding under optimal conditions (Mg^{2+}, Pi or Na^+, ATP, Mg^{2+}) gave straight Scatchard plots for one binding site (cat and human, K_D about 3.5– 5 × 10^{-9}M; guinea pig, K_D about 1.1–1.5 × 10^{-7}M). We have previously shown (3) that the Scatchard plot of ouabain binding to guinea pig cardiac cell membranes under suboptimal conditions (Tyrode solution with 3 mM ATP) was curved, indicating at least two different ouabain binding sites. In the present study, ouabain binding using these suboptimal conditions was further investigated in guinea pig, cat and human cardiac cell membranes.

Scatchard plots of ouabain binding to guinea pig cardiac cell membranes are given in Figure 1. The curved Scatchard plot observed with Tyrode/ATP medium was unchanged when ions other than K^+, for example Ca^2+ (Figure 1A), were omitted. However, omission of K^+ only from the binding medium gave a straight Scatchard plot, for one binding site with an affinity similar to that observed under optimal binding conditions (1.5 × 10^{-7}M; Figure 1A). Further evidence that K^+ is responsible for the induced curvature comes from Figure 1B. Addition of K^+ (1 mM) to the Na^+, ATP, Mg^{2+} medium induced a distinctly curved Scatchard plot.

The K_D-values measured for Tyrode/ATP-supported ouabain binding were about 1–1.5 × 10^{-7}M (high affinity site) and 4–6 × 10^{-6}M (low affinity site). In contracting guinea pig left atria, the EC_{50} for ouabain positive inotropy was 4 × 10^{-7}M while a concentration of 5 × 10^{-6}M inhibited $^{86}Rb^+$-uptake by 50 % (3). Ouabain binding supported by Tyrode solution with 3 mM ATP to cat heart cell membranes (Figure 2A) may be best described by a curved Scatchard plot, indicating at least two different binding sites in this digitalis-sensitive species. Calculations assuming two binding sites gave K_D-values of 3.2 × 10^{-8}M and 9.2 × 10^{-8}M. The K_D for ouabain from the straight Scatchard plot given in Figure 2A for cat cardiac cell membranes was 7.3 × 10^{-8}M. These affinities are similar to the concentrations causing positive inotropy and inhibition of $^{86}Rb^+$-uptake in contracting cat papillary muscles (7). Human cardiac cell membranes gave similar results to cat cardiac cell membranes, in that Tyrode/ATP-supported ouabain binding may be best described by a curved Scatchard plot. The calculated K_D-values, assuming two binding sites, were 2.0 × 10^{-8}M and 1.7 × 10^{-7}M (Figure 2B).

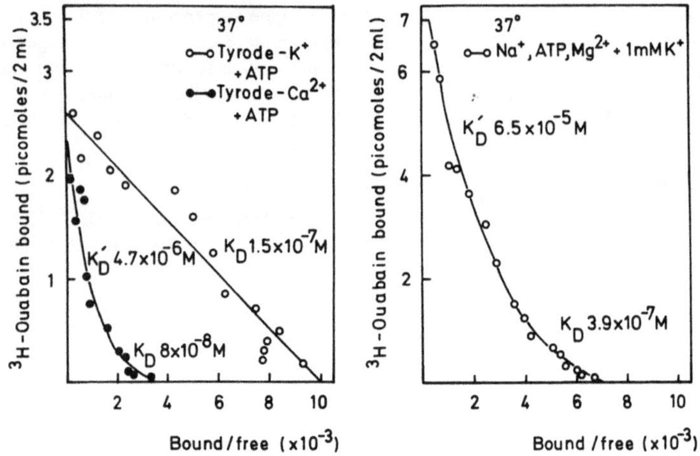

Fig. 1. ^{3}H-Ouabain binding to guinea pig cardiac cell membranes.
Fig. 1A Isolated cell membranes (0.16 mg protein, (Na^+ + K^+)-ATPase activity 0.06 μmol ATP hydrolyzed / min / mg protein at 37 °) were incubated in either Tyrode solution – K^+, with 3 mM ATP or Tyrode solution – Ca^{2+}, with 3 mM ATP, for 2h at 37 °, with increasing concentrations of ^{3}H-ouabain (1×10^{-9}M to 1×10^{-3}M), final volume 2 ml.
Fig. 1B Isolated cell membranes (0.6 mg protein, (Na^+ + K^+)-ATPase activity 0.05 μmol ATP hydrolyzed / min / mg protein at 37 °) were incubated as in Figure 1A using Na^+, ATP, Mg^{2+}-medium with 1 mM K^+.
Bound ouabain was measured after rapid filtration. The K_D-values assuming two binding sites were calculated by the method of Weidemann et al (19).

Discussion

The hypothesis that specific ouabain binding to cell-membrane localized (Na^+ + K^+)-ATPase is responsible for the positive inotropic effects of digitalis can be tested in various systems. Simultaneous measurement of ouabain binding and its consequences on force of contraction and (Na^+ + K^+)-ATPase activity as $^{86}Rb^+$-uptake in contracting cardiac muscle (2, 3) or cultured cardiac cells (4) is necessary for the definition of these sites as receptors. Since the receptor is part of the cell membrane, cardiac cell membrane preparations can be used for further measurements of the effects of specific ouabain binding to (Na^+ + K^+)-ATPase.

For cardiac cell membranes of all species, a stable ^{3}H-ouabain binding could be measured after 60–180 minutes. The non-specific ouabain binding, defined as the binding in the presence of a high concentration (1×10^{-3}M) of unlabelled ouabain, was very low. Further evidence that nearly all of the ouabain binding is specific comes from an examination of the curves for the inhibition of ^{3}H-ouabain binding by various digitalis derivatives (8, 9). As discussed by Laduron (10), the almost total inhibition of ouabain binding by markedly different derivatives indicates that binding except to the specific site is very low. As previously shown (9, 11), specific Mg^{2+}, Pi or Na^+, ATP, Mg^{2+}-supported ouabain binding to beef, cat and human cardiac cell membranes showed one binding site of high affinity.

Simultaneous measurement of ouabain binding and (Na^+ + K^+)-ATPase activity showed concomitant increases in the amount of ouabain bound and decreases in (Na^+ + K^+)-ATPase activity, for beef, cat and human cardiac cell membranes. In contrast, for neonatal rat heart

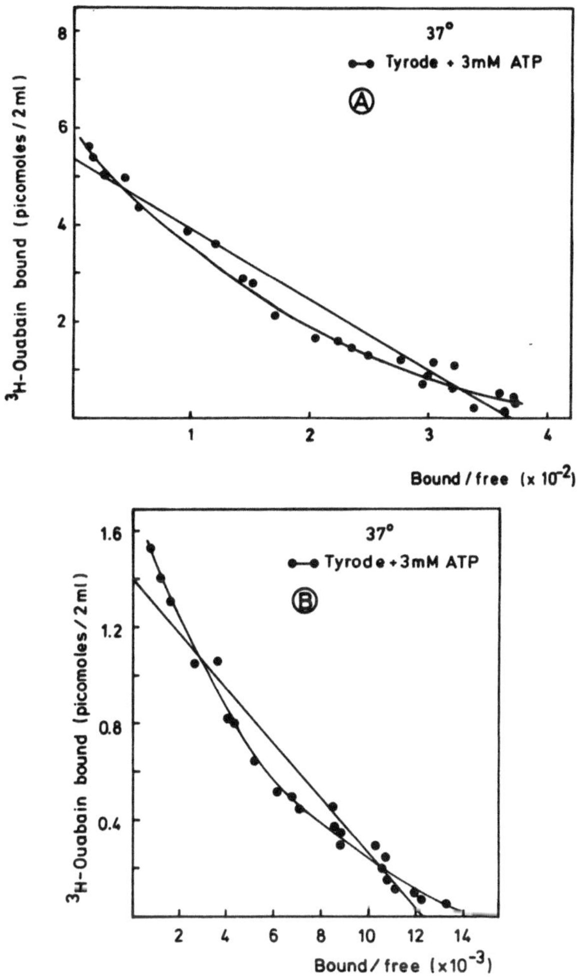

Fig. 2. ^{3}H-Ouabain binding to cat (Figure 2A) and human (Figure 2B) cardiac cell membranes. Isolated cell membranes (cat – 0.18 mg protein, (Na^+ + K^+)-ATPase activity 0.23 μmol ATP hydrolyzed / min / mg protein at 37 °; human – 0.30 mg protein, (Na^+ + K^+)-ATPase activity 0.02 μmol ATP hydrolyzed / min / mg protein at 37 °) were incubated in Tyrode solution with 3 mM ATP for 3h at 37 °, with increasing concentrations of ^{3}H-ouabain (1 × 10^{-9}M to 1 × 10^{-3}M), final volume 2 ml. Bound ouabain was quantitated after rapid filtration. The K_D-values assuming two binding sites were calculated by the method of Weidemann et al (19).

cell membranes, as shown previously for adult rat heart cell membranes (2), ^{3}H-ouabain binding is inhibited at a much lower concentration (IC_{50} = 8 × 10^{-8}M) than the concentration causing 50 % inhibition of (Na^+ + K^+)-ATPase activity (4.8×10^{-5}M).

Schwalb et al (12) gave an IC_{50} of 4.6 × 10^{-5}M for the ouabain inhibition of neonatal rat heart cell membranes. In guinea pig heart cell membranes, ouabain binding also occurred without a corresponding inhibition of (Na^+ + K^+)-ATPase activity but the respective IC_{50}-values differed only by a factor of 3–5 (3). Since the high affinity sites are about 1–20 % of the total number, we may not be able to measure, under the present experimental conditions, an inhibition of ($Na^+ + K^+$)-ATPase activity resulting from binding to the high affinity sites (13, 14).

In the neonatal rat heart, a Scatchard plot of ouabain binding was curved, with only the low affinity site (K_D 1.3 × 10^{-4}M) correlating with the inhibition of ($Na^+ + K^+$)-ATPase (IC_{50} 4.8 × 10^{-5}M). Ouabain binding to guinea pig cardiac cell membranes supported by Tyrode solution with 3 mM ATP, conditions which should more closely approximate experiments with contracting tissue, gave a curved Scatchard plot. Incubation in Tyrode/ATP medium without K^+ (Figure 1A) resulted in a straight Scatchard plot with a K_D-value similar to that under optimal binding conditions. The curvature induced by K^+ in the Scatchard plot of Na^+, ATP, Mg^{2+}-supported binding (Figure 1B) is further evidence that K^+ is responsible for the curvature seen with Tyrode/ATP medium. These results show that K^+ induces an heterogeneity in the ouabain binding sites of guinea pig cardiac cell membranes but do not allow a distinction between two possibilities; a) two distinctly different binding sites, or b) one binding site with a high and low affinity conformation. If the results are calculated for two binding sites, then the high affinity site K_D of 4.7 × 10^{-7}M is similar to the ouabain concentration causing a half-maximal increase in force of contraction in contracting guinea pig left atria (3). In this contracting tissue, higher, toxic ouabain concentrations above 1 × 10^{-6}M are necessary to inhibit $^{86}Rb^+$-uptake – concentrations similar to the K_D of the low affinity site (4 – 6 × 10^{-6}M). These results question the hypothesis that inhibition of ($Na^+ + K^+$)-ATPase is necessary for the positive inotropic effects of digitalis.

Ouabain binding to cardiac cell membranes from the digitalis-sensitive cat and human with Tyrode/ATP medium (Figure 2) is more difficult to interpret. The Scatchard plot may indicate two binding sites with affinities within one order of magnitude. These Scatchard plots could be further examples of K^+-induced heterogeneity of the ouabain binding sites in cardiac cell membranes, as previously shown for the less sensitive guinea pig.

Many workers have studied the modulation by K^+ of the binding of ligands to both the ATP and ouabain binding sites in cell membranes. The K^+-effect on the ATP-binding sites of pig kidney ($Na^+ + K^+$)-ATPase has been investigated by Ottolenghi and Jensen (15). These workers showed that K^+ induced a negative co-operativity in these sites; all binding sites being otherwise identical. In contrast, Hansen (16) showed that addition of K^+ induced homogeneity in the previously inhomogeneous ouabain binding sites of beef brain ($Na^+ + K^+$)-ATPase.

The interactions of K^+, ouabain and dihydroouabain in guinea pig left atria have been studied by Godfraind (17). Low ouabain, but not dihydroouabain, concentrations increased the $^{42}K^+$-uptake. The range of ouabain concentrations giving this stimulation was reduced when the external K^+-concentration was reduced. Further, in guinea pig cardiac cell membranes, these workers showed that K^+ induced a curvature of the Scatchard plot of Na^+, ATP, Mg^{2+} and vanadate-supported ouabain binding (18).

Acknowledgements

We would like to thank Miss A. Reichl and Miss H. Schäffler for skillful technical assistance. These studies were supported by the Deutsche Forschungsgemeinschaft (Er 65/4–3).

References

1. Akera T (1981) Effects of cardiac glycosides on Na^+, K^+-ATPase. In: Handbook of Experimental Pharmacology, vol 56/I, ed Greeff K, Springer Verlag, Berlin, Heidelberg, p 287–336
2. Erdmann E, Philipp G, Scholz H (1980) Cardiac glycoside receptor, ($Na^+ + K^+$)-ATPase activity and force of contraction in rat heart. Biochem Pharmacol 29:3219–3222

3. Brown L, Werdan K, Erdmann E (1983) Consequences of specific ^{3}H-ouabain binding to guinea pig left atria and cardiac cell membranes. Biochem Pharmacol 32:423–435
4. Werdan K, Zwißler B, Wagenknecht B, Krawietz W, Erdmann E (1983) Quantitative correlation of cardiac glycoside binding to its receptor and inhibition of the sodium pump in chicken heart cells in culture. Biochem Pharmacol 32:757–760
5. Schoner W, von Ilberg C, Kramer R, Seubert W (1967) On the mechanism of adenosine triphosphatase. 1. Purification and properties of a Na^+- and K^+-activated ATPase from ox brain. Eur J Biochem 1:334–343
6. Lowry OH, Rosebrough NJ, Farr AL, Randall RJ (1951) Protein measurement with the Folin phenol reagent. J Biol Chem 193:265–275
7. Erdmann E, Philipp G, Scholz H (1981) Evidence for two receptors for cardiac glycosides in the heart. In: Godfraind T, Meyer P, eds Cell membrane in function and dysfunction of vascular tissue. Elsevier North-Holland, Amsterdam, p 76–83
8. Brown L, Erdmann E, Thomas R (1983) Digitalis structure-activity relationship analyses: conclusions from indirect binding studies with cardiac ($Na^+ + K^+$)-ATPase. Biochem Pharmacol 32:2767–2774
9. Brown L, Erdmann E (1984) Comparison of the affinity of human, beef and cat heart ($Na^+ + K^+$)-ATPase for different digitalis derivatives Arzneim-Forsch, in press
10. Laduron P (1983) More binding, more fancy. Trends in Pharmacological Sciences, 333–334
11. Brown L, Erdmann E (1983) The cardiac glycoside-receptor system in the human heart. Eur Heart J 4 (Suppl A):61–65
12. Schwalb H, Dickstein Y, Heller M (1982) Interactions of cardiac glycosides with cardiac cells III. Alterations in the sensitivity of ($Na^+ + K^+$)-ATPase to inhibition by ouabain in rat hearts. Biochim Biophys Acta 689:241–248
13. Adams RJ, Schwartz A, Grupp G, Grupp I, Lee SW, Wallick ET, Powell T, Twist VW, Gathiram P (1982) High-affinity binding site and low-dose positive inotropic effect in rat myocardium. Nature 296: 167–169
14. Lelievre LG, Mansier P, Charlemagne D, Swynghedauw B (1984) Effects of calcium on the heterogeneity of the Na^+, K^+-ATPase forms in rat heart. Basic Res Cardiol, this issue
15. Ottolenghi P, Jensen J (1983) The K^+-induced apparent heterogeneity of high-affinity nucleotide-binding sites in ($Na^+ + K^+$)-ATPase can only be due to the oligomeric structure of the enzyme. Biochim Biophys Acta: 727:89–100
16. Hansen O (1976) Non-uniform populations of g-strophanthin binding sites of ($Na^+ + K^+$)-activated ATPase. Apparent conversion to uniformity by K^+. Biochim Biophys Acta 433:383–392
17. Godfraind T (1981) Stimulation and inhibition of the Na^+, K^+-pump by cardiac glycosides. In: Handbook of Experimental Pharmacology, vol 56/I, ed Greeff K, Springer Verlag, Berlin, Heidelberg, p 381–393
18. Godfraind T, de Pover A, Tona Lutete DN (1980) Identification with potassium and vanadate of two classes of specific ouabain binding sites in a ($Na^+ + K^+$)-ATPase preparation from the guinea pig heart. Biochem Pharmacol 29:1195–1199
19. Weidemann MJ, Erdelt H, Klingenberg M (1970) Adenine nucleotide translocation of mitochondria. Eur J Biochem 16:313–335

Authors' address:

Dr. Lindsay Brown, Medizinische Klinik I der Universität, Klinikum Großhadern, Marchioninistr. 15, 8000 München 70

Contractility of isolated bovine ventricular myocytes is enhanced by intracellular injection of cardioactive glycosides. Evidence for an intracellular mode of action

G. Isenberg

II. Physiologisches Institut, Universität des Saarlandes, Homburg (FRG)

Summary

The contractions of isolated bovine left ventricular myocytes were evaluated by optically measuring the extent of unloaded shortening (ES), the maximal rate of shortening (MRS) and the maximal rate of re-lengthening (MRL).

Ouabain, digoxin or digitoxin were intracellularly injected by 2 sec long pressure pulses via the microelectrodes. Their i.c. concentration was estimated to be 2–5 nM. Within 1–4 min after the injection, ES, MRS and MRL increased by more than 2fold. The contractility renormalized within the following 20 min. Injection of solutions without glycosides did not increase the contractility.

An interaction of the injected glycoside with the e.c. ouabain receptor could be largely excluded because a) the amount of the released glycoside was too small for e.c. effects, b) 500 nM e.c. antidigoxin, c) 20 mM $[K]_o$ or d) covalent binding of digoxin to HSA did not prevent the increase in contractility due to the i.c. injections.

Since contractility also increased when the injections were performed at Na-free conditions, $[Na]_i$-load is not necessary for the effect of i.c. glycosides. The increased contractility due to the injected glycosides was not observed when the contractility prior to the injection was already potentiated, e.g. by >3.6 mM $[Ca]_o$ or by stimulation at frequencies >1.25 Hz.

The results are interpreted by the hypothesis that the i.c. glycosides facilitate the release of activator calcium from the SR. The possible i.c. modes of action are discussed as well as the idea that e.c. applied glycosides internalize and mediate inotropy via the i.c. mechanism.

Key words: inotropy – cardioactive glycosides – isolated myocyte – intracellular injection

Introduction

The inotropic effect of cardioactive glycosides is usually explained by the "sodium lag hypothesis". This hypothesis postulates the following sequence of events: 1) the glycosides specifically bind to an extracellular (e.c.) receptor on the Na,K-ATPase. 2) As a result of inhibition of the Na,K-ATPase ("pump inhibition"), $[Na]_i$ increases ($[Na]_i$-load) 3) Since transsarcolemmal Na- and Ca-gradients are coupled via the Na,Ca exchange, $[Na]_i$load leads to $[Ca]_i$ load. 4) The extra $[Ca]_i$ is taken up by intracellular (i.c.) stores, probably the sarcoplasmic reticulum (SR). 5. Filled stores release more activator calcium thereby resulting in inotropy. All of the above five steps are well documented (ct. ref. Wasserstrom et al., 1983) and I do not intend to question them. The topic of this contribution is to question whether "the sodium lag" is the only possible mechanism by which cardioactive glycosides can increase the contractility, or whether or not other mechanisms exist.

Cardiac cells can take up glycosides from the extracellular space ("internalization") and accumulate them in the microsomal fraction (Dutta et al., 1968, Fricke et al., 1969; Dutta &

Marks, 1972; Park & Vincenzi, 1975; Fricke 1978). Because the inotropy correlates with the internalization, a "second" inotropic mechanism mediated by an intracellular (i.c.) digitalis receptor has been suggested. Hess & Müller (1982) tested the concept of the i.c. inotropic receptor by applying digoxin to bovine ventricular trabeculae (the e.c.s. filled with antidigoxin) via the cut end. Under these conditions they could not demonstrate an increase in contractility. Before accepting their negative result as definite evidence against an i.c. digitalis receptor that mediates inotropy, one should consider that the cut end method (Weingart, 1974) applies the drug with steep gradients over the length of the trabecula (Hess & Müller, 1982: Fig. 4). Thus, a possible inotropic effect could have remained undetected because a small region with inotropy could have worked against the compliance of the major part of the trabecula which was either unmodified or intoxicated.

Due to those uncertainties, it might be necessary to re-investigate possible i.c. effects of cardiac glycosides. The isolated ventricular myocyte provides a model where the drugs can directly be applied by intracellular injection. Problems of cell-to-cell diffusion do not exist. In addition, due to the small dimensions of the single cell, the drug should distribute rapidly and more homogenously. Moreover, contractility can be recorded from that same cell into which the drug was injected.

Special problems arise from the inability to attach a transducer to the single myocyte for force measurements. The contractile state of the unloaded cell was characterized by determining the extent and rate of shortening of the sarcomeres. It was found that both extent (ES) and maximal rate of shortening (MRS) increase after the i.c. injection of the glycosides ouabain, digoxin, and digitoxin. Because the term "inotropy" does not apply (inos = force), I have called the enhanced contractility "contractropy" defined as increase in ES and MRS. On p. 13 I will discuss that contractropy and inotropy are directly related.

Methods

The procedure of cell isolation has been published elsewhere in detail (Isenberg & Klöckner, 1982). Briefly, chunks of adult bovine left ventricular tissue were incubated in a medium containing hyaluronidase (0.5 g/l) and collagenase (0.5 g/l) as well as 30 μM $CaCl_2$. The isolated cells were stored in a KB-medium to become Ca-tolerant. For the experiment, some of these cells were transferred to a 1 ml chamber, where they were continuously superfused with a Tyrode solution composed of 150 mM NaCl, 5.4 mM KCl, 1.8 mM $CaCl_2$, 2 mM $MgCl_2$, 10 mM glucose, 5 mM Hepes (adjusted with NaOH to pH 7.4). The temperature was 35 °C.

Glass microelectrodes were filled with a 150 mM KCl solution buffered with 10 mM MOPS/KOH to pH 7.2. They had resistances of about 60 MOhm suggesting tip diameters of about 0.5 μm. The electrodes were connected to an input amplifier that allows stimulation through the voltage-recording electrode (Dreyer & Peper, 1974). After impalement, the cell hang on to the microelectrode, and both were lifted from the bottom of the chamber by about 50 μm. In response to i.c. stimuli (0.2 Hz), the myocyte contracted by moving both cell edges towards the microelectrode tip as the fix point. This shortening and re-lengthening was continuously monitored on a TV-camera-tape system (Isenberg, 1982). On the monitor, the moving cell edge lightened or shadowed an array of 50 photodiodes thereby resulting in an analog signal for the shortening and re-lenghtening of the myocyte. The signal was filtered at 10 Hz and recorded together with its first derivative on a BRUSH pen writer. Off line, the records were calibrated in terms of the average sarcomere length that was evaluated from single images of the TV tape (for details see Isenberg, 1982, Fig. 1). The sarcomeres shortened from a maximum diastolic length (SL_d) to a minimum systolic length (SL_s) within about 300 ms (TTP). The extent of shortening (ES) was calculated according to $(Sl_d\text{-}SL_s)/SL_d$. In the example of Fig. 2, SL_d is 1.85 μm, SL_s 1.69 μm, and one calculates an ES of 8.6%. The rate of shortening and re-lengthening of the average sarcomere was estimated by dividing the change in sarcomere length by the 20 ms interval between consecutive semi-images (50 Hz TV system). Using the above figures, one calculated for maximum rate of shortening (MRS) −1 μm/s and for the maximum rate of re-lengthening (MRL) 0.95 μm/s.

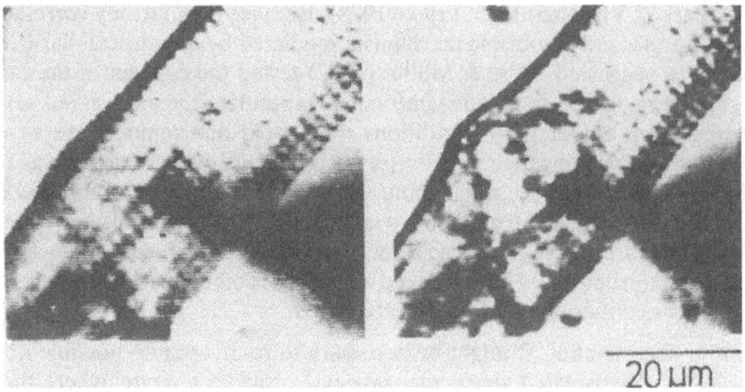

Fig. 1. Central part of a bovine ventricular myocyte with an impaled microelectrode; volume changes due to pressure injection. Single images from the TV tape. Left: before, right: after injection of about 1 pl of the filling solution.
The volume to be injected was calibrated before impalement; with the tip placed in oil, the pressure ejected a drop whose diameter was measured (see Isenberg, 1977). Inside the cell the injection produced a local swelling. Due to this swelling the upper part of the cell runs out of focus changing to a white image. The swelling disappeared within 20 s suggesting that the injected 1 pl distributed over the cell volume of 50 pl, diluting the i.c. concentrations correspondingly.

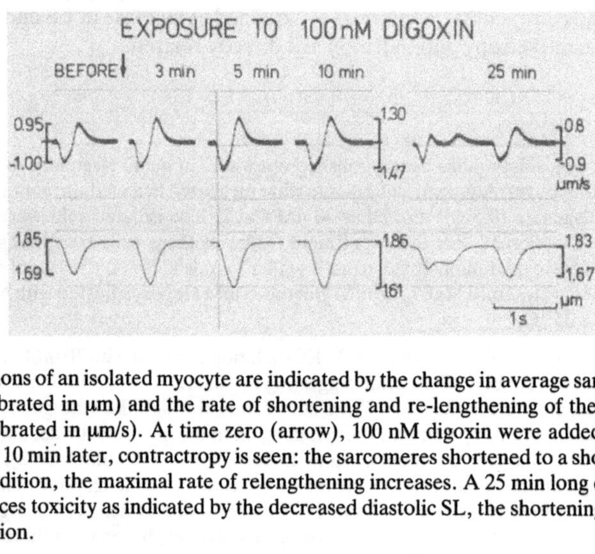

Fig. 2. Contractions of an isolated myocyte are indicated by the change in average sarcomere length (SL, lower traces calibrated in µm) and the rate of shortening and re-lengthening of the sarcomere (upper, noisy traces, calibrated in µm/s). At time zero (arrow), 100 nM digoxin were added to the superfusing Tyrode solution. 10 min later, contractropy is seen: the sarcomeres shortened to a shorter systolic SL at a faster rate. In addition, the maximal rate of relengthening increases. A 25 min long exposure to 100 nM e.c. digoxin induces toxicity as indicated by the decreased diastolic SL, the shortening to greater SL, and the aftercontraction.

Limitations of the method. The TV system delivers a maximum of 50 (semi-)images per second, therefore the "true" SL_s and the "true" rates will be underestimated. Often, the base line of the pen recordings drifted because of stray light, changes in the meniscus surrounding the microelectrode, air bubbles, or debris floating in the medium. Thus, the pen record was frequently re-calibrated from the single images of the TV tape.

For the i.c. injection an air pressure pulse (4 bar) was applied to the open end of the glass pipette via a special holder (see Isenberg, 1979). Occasionally, the intracellular pressure injections broke the seal of the cell membrane to the glass tip, as a consequence, the membrane depolarized and the AP decreased in its amplitude and duration. Normally, those events did not occur indicating the absence of a leak between intra- and extracellular space.

The cardiac glycosides – ouabain, digoxin, or digitoxin – were added to the filling electrolyte to give a final concentration of 100 nM. To chelate contaminating calcium, 20 μM K_2EGTA were added (see. p. 6). The volume to be injected was calibrated prior to the experiment with the tip placed in oil where the pressure ejected droplets of a radius between 2 and 5 μm (see Isenberg 1977). With the micropipette tip intracellularly, the same pressure pulse was applied; in addition, the injected volume was monitored by the cell swelling (recorded with the TV system, see Fig. 1.). A drop of 5 μm radius has a volume of 0.5 pl. Distributed over the cell volume of about 50 pl, the volume fraction is about 1%. Assuming that the free water constitutes more that 50% of the cell (Page, 1978) the injected glycoside will be diluted 50fold to an "effective" i.c. concentration of approx. 2 nM. The local cell swelling disappeared within 10–20 sec, probably the "injectans" and the drug spread out by streaming. Diffusion should distribute the glycoside homogenously within less than 5 min (calculated for a distance of 100 μm with $D = 8.5 \cdot 10^{-8} cm^2 \cdot s$ from Hess & Müller 1982, for intra- and intercellular diffusion of ^{3}H-digoxin).

The anti-digoxin (Fab-fragment with a molecular weight of 60,000) as well as the digoxin covalently bound to human serum albumin (7 digoxin molecules per HSA, molecular weight 10,600 per digoxin molecule) were kindly provided by Dr. W. Riesen, Institut für Tumorforschung, University of Bern, Switzerland.

Results

1. Contractropy due to e.c. applied glycosides

Before i.c. injection, the glycosides were conventionally applied to the bath in order to test whether or not the unloaded shortening of the isolated myocytes can be used as a model. Fig. 2 gives the result which is typical for 5 other cells. When the cell was stimulated at 0.2 Hz and 100 nM digoxin were added to the Tyrode solution, within 10 min the following "contractrope" events were recorded: With an unchanged TTP, the systole shortened the SL to 1.61 instead of 1.69 um. Thus, the extent of shortening (ES) increased by a factor of 1.56 from 8.8 to 13.4%. The maximal rate of shortening (MRS) increased from –1 μm/s to –1.47 μm/s. The maximal rate of re-lengthening (MRL) increased from 0.95 μm/s to 1.3 μm/s. With longer exposure (25 min), toxic effects were indicated by shortening of the SL_d, prolonged TTP, shortening to longer SL_s, as well as by aftercontractions and afterdepolarizations, eventually followed by triggered automaticity (for guinea pig papillary muscles compare Reiter, 1962). In Tyrode solution containing 3.6 instead of 1.8 mM $CaCl_2$, the glycosides failed to induce contractropy (n = 4), and only toxic effects were observed. The contractrope effect strongly depended on the frequency of stimulation: maximal effectiveness at 0.1 Hz and a "ceiling off" at 1 Hz were observed (compare Koch-Weser & Blinks, 1962, 1963).

When, after a 10 min exposure to 100 nM digoxin, the drug was washed out, the contractility re-normalized within about 5 min. In the presence of 100 nM digoxin, contractility could be re-normalized by 500 nM anti-digoxin within 3 min. Also, increasing the $[KCl]_o$ from 5.4 mM to 20 mM nearly abolished the contractropy in the presence of 100 nM digoxin. When 100 nM digoxin was added to a sodium free Tyrode solution (NaCl isoosmotically replaced ty 290 mM taurine), no contractropy was seen (observed up to 40 min). (For multicellular preparations, the dependence of inotropy on $[K]_o$ and $[Na]_o$ has been described e.g. by Fricke & Klaus, 1971, or Prindle et al., 1971.)

In summary, the results resemble the inotropic effects reported in multicellular preparations such as papillary muscles or trabeculae. The greater ES and MRS will be considered as counterpart to the increase in the force of contraction.

2. *Contractropy by i.c. injected glycosides*

Fig. 3 shows contractions before, during and after the i.c. injection of 2 nM ouabain. Before injection, the cell contracted weakly (ES = 4%, MRS = –0.5 µm/s, MRL = 0.3 µm/s). Immediately after injection, the cell contractions were stronger. Half a minute after injection, the extent of shortening was 11%, i.e. nearly 3 fold greater than before injection (4%). The sarcomeres shortened (–0.85 µm/s instead of –0.5 µm/s) and also re-lengthened faster (0.75 µm/s instead of 3 µm/s).

The injected solution induced a spontaneous irregular "twiggling" of groups of about 8 sarcomeres. The amplitude of this "twiggling" peaked within 10–30 sec and nearly disappeard within another min (see the noise in Figs. 3, 4). Twiggling also occurred when the injectans was free of the glycoside, and when it contained 20 µM EGTA (see below). The twiggling was not observed, when chloride free solutions were injected. Therefore, it might be related to the "depolarization induced calcium release" of the sarcoplasmic reticulum (Endo, 1977). Because the twiggling was an event independent of the contractropy induced by the i.c. injected glycosides, it will not be further discussed.

The surprisingly fast onset of the contractropy could suggest that the underlying mechanism does not involve the injected glycoside. This possibility was tested by injecting the electrolyte without the glycoside. The cells responded to those injections with a 30 sec long "twiggling" (see above). In addition, a small transient contractropy increased the ES from 7.2 to 9%, the MRS from –1.5 to –2 µm/s, and the MRL from 1.2 to 1.5 µm/s (4 cells). This contractropy peaked within 20 s and disappeared within the next min. When 20 µM K_2EGTA were added to the injectans, the cells no longer responded with contractropy but with slightly depressed contractions. This depressant effect lasted for about 1 min (see Figs. 4, 5). The finding suggests that the small "immediate contractropy" results from the Ca-contamination of the injectans. To prevent it, all the subsequent injections were performed with 20 µM EGTA in the injectans (see Method, p 4).

The contractropy elicited by injecting a solution that contained 20 µM EGTA and 0.1 µM digoxin is shown in Fig. 4. Just after the injection, the cell responded with depressed

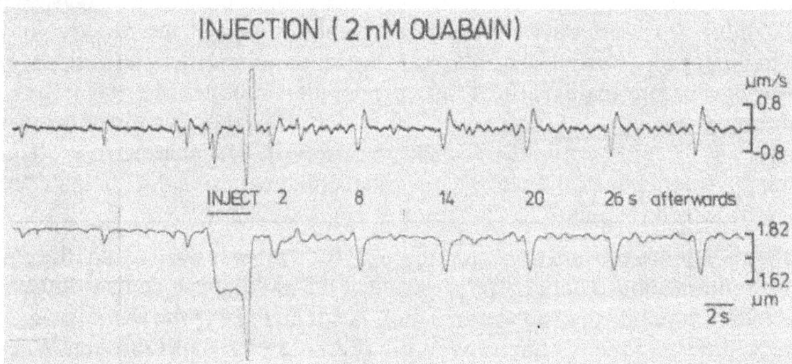

Fig. 3. Contractropy recorded from an isolated myocyte injected with 0.3 pl of a solution composed of 150 mM KCl, 10 mM MOPS/KOH buffer (pH 7.2) and 100 nM ouabain. I.c., the ouabain will be diluted to about 2 nM. During the pressure (4 bar for 1.5 s, label "inject"), tip and cell moved by about 20 µm but repositioned afterwards. After the injection, "contractropy" develops: the extent of shortening (lower row) as well as the rate of shortening and of re-lengthening (upper row) increase. The "twiggling" (noisy deflections during diastole) and a transient minor part of the contractropy were also seen in control experiments injecting solutions without glycoside.

contractility and "twiggling". In the subsequent minute, contractility increased. The sarcomeres shortened from a constant SL_d to a shorter SL_s (1.63 instead of 1.78 um). Comparing the contractions before and 1 min after injection, the ES increased from 4.3% to 11.9%. The cell shortened faster, the MRS changed from –0.25 to –1 μm/s, and the MRL from 0.2 to 1.0 μm/s.

Fig. 7 gives an example of contractions recorded with an expanded time scale. Injecting i.c. 4 nM digoxin evoked a contractropy that peaked within about 4 min. Similar as in the experiment of Fig. 4, the cell in Fig. 6 responded to the injection with an increase in ES (3.8 to 9.3%), in MRS (–0.8 μm/s to –2.1 μm/s), and in MRL (0.5 to 2.9 μm/s).

Mean values and standard errors of the measured contractile parameters were averaged from 12 cells before and after injection at peak contractropy, the i.c. concentrations of ouabain (n = 3), digoxin (n = 6) and digitoxin (n = 3) being similar (2–4 nM). The diastolic SL did not change significantly (1.85 ± 0.04 μm before, 1.84 ± 0.06 μm after injection). The systolic SL changed significantly from 1.73 ± 0.09 to 1.59 ± 0.06 μm. The ES increased from 4.5 ± 0.9% to 11.1 ± 0.7%. The TTP increased slightly from 280 ± 30 to 330 ± 70 ms. The MRS increased from 0.55 ± 0.1 μm/s to 1.08 ± 0.1 μm/s. The MRL increased from 0.4 ± 0.1

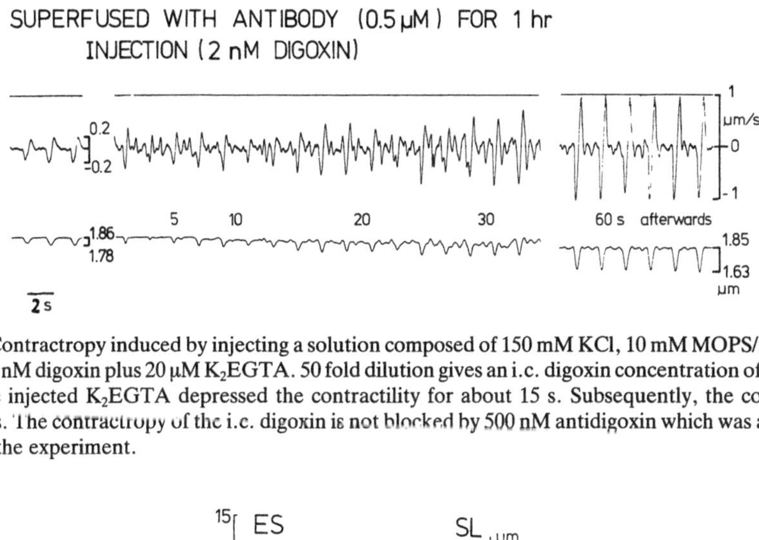

Fig. 4. Contractropy induced by injecting a solution composed of 150 mM KCl, 10 mM MOPS/KOH (pH 7.2), 100 nM digoxin plus 20 μM K_2EGTA. 50 fold dilution gives an i.c. digoxin concentration of approx. 2 nM. The injected K_2EGTA depressed the contractility for about 15 s. Subsequently, the contractility increases. The contractropy of the i.c. digoxin is not blocked by 500 nM antidigoxin which was added 1 hr prior to the experiment.

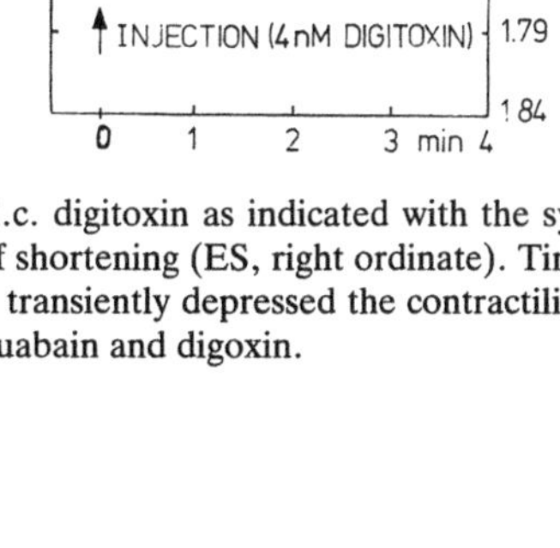

Fig. 5. Contractropy by 4 nM i.c. digitoxin as indicated with the systolic sarcomere length (SL, right ordinate) and with the extent of shortening (ES, right ordinate). Time course of the development. The EGTA-content of the injectans transiently depressed the contractility. Note: a similar time course was recorded also for i.c. injected ouabain and digoxin.

μm/s to 1.3 ± 0.3 μm/s. Comparing all these changes, the maximum rate of re-lengthening (MRL) seems to be the most sensitive parameter. Among the glycosides ouabain, digoxin, and digitoxin, no significant differences could be determined ($p = 0.2$).

The onset of the contractropy is illustrated in Fig. 5 for a digitoxin injection. Usually, the contractropy peaked within 3–5 min after the injection of ouabain, digoxin or digitoxin. Independent of the type of the injected glycoside, the contractropy developed with a half time of 70 ± 15 sec (n = 12); significant differences among ouabain, digoxin, or digitoxin could not be evaluated.

Reversibility: The contractropy decayed from the maximum (4 min in Fig. 7) slowly with time, reaching the contractile state before injection within 20–30 min. The transient nature of the contractropy suggests that the i.c. injected glycoside can slowly leave the cell. When contractility had re-normalized, a second injection of the cardioactive glycoside could evoke a similar contractropy as the first one. When the second injection was performed before the effects of the first injection had disappeared, cumulative effects were seen.

3. The contractropy results from the i.c. glycoside

One could argue that, although the glycosides were injected intracellularly, they could cross the sarcolemma ("leak" trough the membrane) and interact with the extracellular ouabain receptor. If such was the case then the contractropy would be attributed not to an i.c. but to an e.c. glycoside effect. This possibility was excluded with the following experiments:

a) The putative e.c. glycoside concentration should be (much) lower than 100 nM in the injectans because the drug leaves the electrode only during the 1–2 sec long pressure pulse, and because it will be diluted and washed away by the superfusate. Thus, a comparison of the i.c. effects with 100 nM e.c. glycoside should be more than appropriate. When 100 nM digoxin or ouabain were added to the bath for a period of 10 seconds, no contractrope effects were observed. When concentrations of 100 nM were e.c. applied for 10 min, it enhanced the ES from 8 to 12% (see Fig. 2). Thus, the contractropy of a 10 min exposure to 100 nM e.c. digoxin is smaller than the contractropy induced by a 2 sec i.c. injection of 2–4 nM digoxin. Regarding the e.c. ouabain, a 20 sec exposure to 100 nM did not modify the contractions. A 10 min application of 100 nM e.c. ouabain increased the ES from 9 to 11% (n = 4). When 100 nM ouabain were e.c. administered, no contractropy was seen within 20 min (n = 3). Thus, one concludes that glycosides added to the bath in 50fold greater concentrations and/or for 200fold longer times (than applied i.c.) can not mimic the contractropy due to the injected i.c. glycosides. Therefore, an explanation based on the leak of the glycoside through the membrane, followed by the e.c. drug-receptor interaction seems to be unlikely.

As an additional control experiment, a solution containing 1 μM adrenaline instead of the glycoside was i.c. injected. (Adrenaline permeates through the lipid bilayer with a similar rate to ouabain.) The injection of adrenaline did not induce contractropy. Because even 20 nM adrenaline e.c. induces a clear increase in the ES, the negative result argues against a significant "leak" of the injected drug.

b) Glycosides i.c. injected but hypothetically leaking into the e.c.s. can be trapped by antibodies. In control experiments, 500 nM e.c. antidigoxin abolished the contractropy induced by 100 nM e.c. digoxin (given 10 min in advance) within 4–5 min (n = 3, see also Smith et al., 1971; Hess & Müller, 1982). Adding 100 nM e.c. digoxin to a Tyrode solution containing 500 nM e.c. antidigoxin did not change the contractility. Regarding the i.c. injection experiments, the cells were exposed to 500 nM e.c. antidigoxin for a period of 1 hr prior to the i.c. injection. (The long exposure should allow the antidigoxin to diffuse into the system of the transversal tubuli.) The e.c. antidigoxin did not prevent or attenuate the contractropy induced by i.c. injections of 2–4 nM digoxin (n = 5, see Fig. 4). The ES, MRS and MRL measured after injections with (n = 5) and without (n = 6) the e.c. antidigoxin did not significantly differ (p = 0.2). Regarding the contractropy mediated by digoxin leaking through the membrane and acting from the e.c.s. via the extracellular ouabain receptor, the antidigoxin should have at least attenuated the effects of the i.c. injected digoxin. The lack of the effect of antidigoxin suggests that the i.c. injected glycoside can induce contractropy via a receptor accessible from the inside of the cell.

c) Digoxin can be covalently bound to human serum albumin. The macromolecule is unable to cross the membrane. Smith et al. (1972) applied the covalently bound digoxin e.c. to the bath and observed that the conjugates neither inhibited the Na,K-ATPhase nor induced inotropy. Small effects were attributed to a 0.1–1% contamination with non-bound glycosides. Provided the same degree of contamination holds true for the present experiments, the injectans may contain 0.1–1 nM of free digoxin. When such a digoxin concentration was e.c. applied to the bath, no contractropy was induced. When i.c. injected, the macromolecule should stay inside the cell. The i.c. injection of 10 nM covalently bound digoxin induced contractropy (Fig. 6): within 5 min, it more than doubled the ES (from 12.5 to 28%), increased the MRS 2.3fold (from –0.9 to –2.1 μm/s), and the MRL 3.2fold (from 0.9 to 2.9 μm/s). Aftercontractions indicate that the i.c. injection also induced toxic effects.

The result of Fig. 6 was reproduced 4 times, and all 5 cells responded to the injection of digoxin covalently bound to human serum albumin with a strong contractropy. The results suggest that the i.c. injected drug binds to a receptor that has diffusional access from the cytosol. It further suggests that the albumin does not sterically hinder the digoxin-receptor interaction.

d) Experiments in the presence of 20 mM $[K]_o$. Elevated $[K]_o$ is known to antagonize the inotropic and toxic effects of cardioactive glycosides (ct. ref. Lee & Klaus, 1971), probably by reducing the affinity of the e.c. ouabain receptor (ct. ref. Fricke & Klaus, 1971; Prindle et al., 1971). Thus, in the presence of 100 nM e.c. digoxin (10 min), elevating $[K]_o$ from 5.4 to 20 mM abolished the digoxin induced contractropy within 5 min (n = 3), see p. 4. At 20 mM $[K]_o$, e.c. application of 100 nM digoxin (n = 3) or digitoxin (n = 4) did not induce contractropy. In contrast to its antagonism of the e.c. effects of glycosides, 20 mM $[KCl]_o$ did not prevent or reduce the contractropy caused by i.c. injection of 3–5 nM digoxin (n = 3) or digitoxin (n = 5).

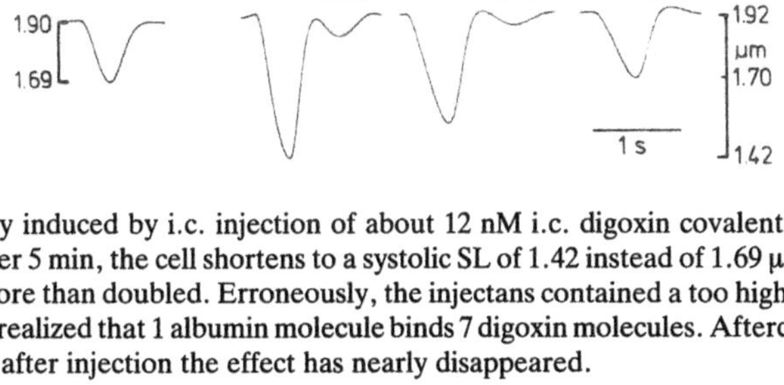

Fig. 6. Contractropy induced by i.c. injection of about 12 nM i.c. digoxin covalently bound to human serum albumin. After 5 min, the cell shortens to a systolic SL of 1.42 instead of 1.69 μm. Thus, the extent of shortening has more than doubled. Erroneously, the injectans contained a too high digoxin concentration since it was not realized that 1 albumin molecule binds 7 digoxin molecules. Aftercontractions suggest toxicity. Note: 1 hr after injection the effect has nearly disappeared.

In Fig. 7, the injection of 4 nM digoxin induced within 4 min the following effects: the cell shortened to a SL_s of 1.45 instead of 1.7 μm which corresponds to a 2.6fold increase in the ES from 8 to 21%. The MRS increased 3fold from –0.3 to –0.9 μm/s, and the MRL increased 5.5fold from 0.2 to 1.1 μm/s. Fig. 9A shows the contractropy mediated by an injection of 4 nM i.c. digitoxin in the presence of 20 mM $[K]_o$. Evaluated as an example for a stimulation at 10 sec intervals, SL_s falls from 1.78 (control) to 1.56 μm corresponding a 3.7fold increase in ES. MRS increased 3fold from 0.35 to 1.2 μm/s, and MRL 4.3fold from 0.35 to 1.5 μm/s. In comparing the contractropy induced by i.c. injections among cells superfused with solutions containing 5.4 mM $[K]_o$ (n = 12) and those superfused with media containing 20 mM $[K]_o$, no significant differences could be detected (p = 0.2). Thus, an interaction of the i.c. glycoside with the $[K]_o$ sensitive e.c. ouabain receptor is unlikely.

4. Contractropy due to i.c. glycosides does not require $[Na]_i$-load

Myocytes superfused for 30 min with a medium containing no sodium and 20 mM KCl responded with slow action potentials and contractions that started from nearly normal diastolic sarcomere lengths (Fig. 8). ES and MRS were comparable to the values in sodium containing media. However, the sarcomeres re-lengthened very slowly, the MRL was 0.1 μm/s or less. Probably, the decay of activator calcium is slowed when Na-free media supresses the Na-Ca exchange (see below).

Five min after i.c. injection of 6 nM ouabain, the cell responded with a clear contractropy (Fig. 8). The sarcomeres shortened to 1.47 instead of 1.64 μm which corresponds to a doubling of the ES (from 11 to 20.5%). In addition, the SL_s was achieved in a slightly shorter time (340 instead of 390 ms). MRS increased about 3fold (from 1.1 to 3.2 μm/s). The most prominent effect of the i.c. ouabain injection was to speed up the relaxation process; the sarcomeres re-

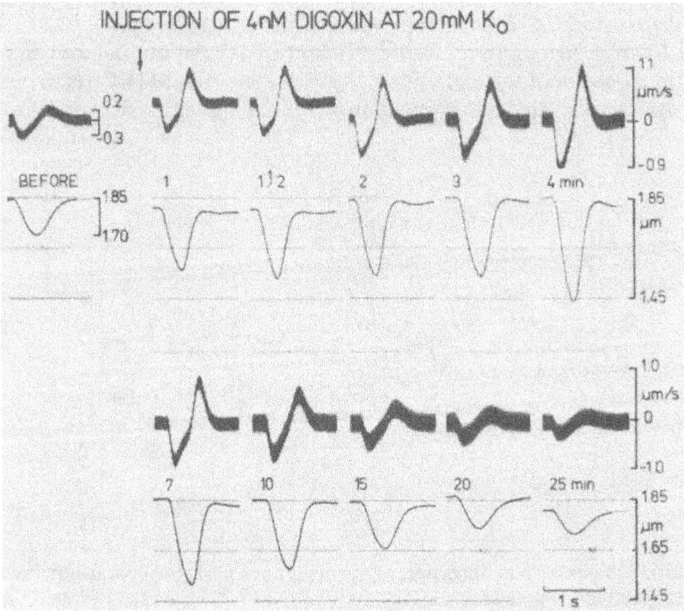

Fig. 7. Contractropy evoked by i.c. injection of 4 nM digoxin in presence of 20 mM KCl. The high $[K]_o$ does not block the contractropy which peaks within 4 min and disappears within 20 min.

lengthened to the diastolic 1.85 μm within 350 ms (after the systole), before the injection within such a period no re-lenthening was seen at all. MRL increased 6fold from 0.5 to 3.3 μm/s. Attributing the faster re-lengthening to a faster decline of the i.c. activator calcium ("activation dependent relaxation" according to Brutsaert et al., 1978), the results suggest that the i.c. glycoside can enhance the rate of the calcium uptake from the cytosol into the i.c. calcium stores.

Contractropy in Na-free media was induced by 2 digoxin injections and 4 ouabain injections, only 1 ouabain injection failed to induce contractropy. After 30 min in Na-free media, $[Na]_i$ is only 1.5 mM and the sodium pump is arrested (Sheu et al., 1980). Therefore, it is unlikely that the contractropy induced by ouabain injections results from an altered ATPase activity controlling the calcium binding of neighboured phosphatidylserine molecules (ct. ref. Lüllmann & Peters, 1981). Also, one can exclude the i.c. sodium load as causal event because the medium in the e.c.s. is sodium-free. Thus, this type of experiment indicates that i.c. glycosides can induce contractropy without involving Na,K-ATPase or $[Na]_i$.

5. *Dependence on the contractile state before injection*

The i.c. injection of cardioactive glycosides can induce contractropy only in cells that do not already "optimally" contract. Vice versa, the contractrope effects are greater when the contractions prior to the injection were weak. Two examples may clarify the situation:

a) Dependence on the stimulation interval. Like the contractile force of multicellular papillary muscles or trabeculae (Koch-Weser & Blinks, 1962, 1963), the unloaded shortening of the isolated myocyte depends on the stimulation interval (Fig. 9, see also Isenberg, 1982): ES, MRS and MRL achieve a minimum for 20 s long intervals. They moderately increase when the interval is longer (Fig. 9, control, increase of the curves to the right). All 3 parameters strongly increase when the intervals are shortened, or correspondingly, when the

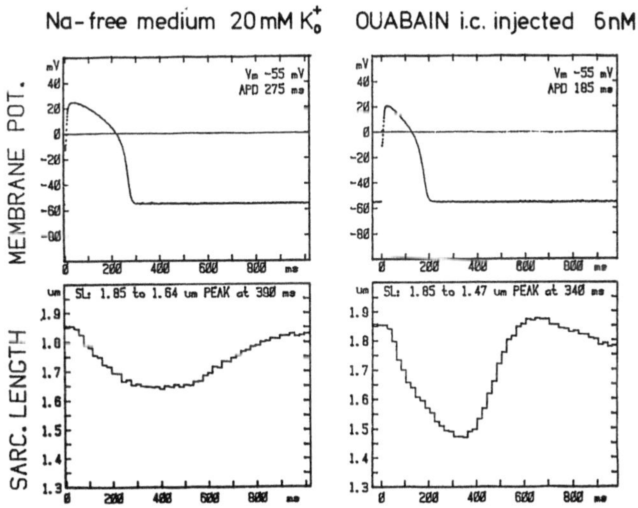

Fig. 8. Contractropy in absence of $[Na]_o$ by i.c. injection of 6 nM ouabain. Slow action potentials (top) and contractions (below) from a cell superfused with a Na-free medium 30 min prior and during the experiment. The tracings on the right were obtained when the contractropy peaked at 5 min after the injection. In the Na-free medium, 150 mM NaCl was isoosmotically replaced by 290 mM taurine, 10 mM Tris/Hepes buffered the medium to pH 7.4.

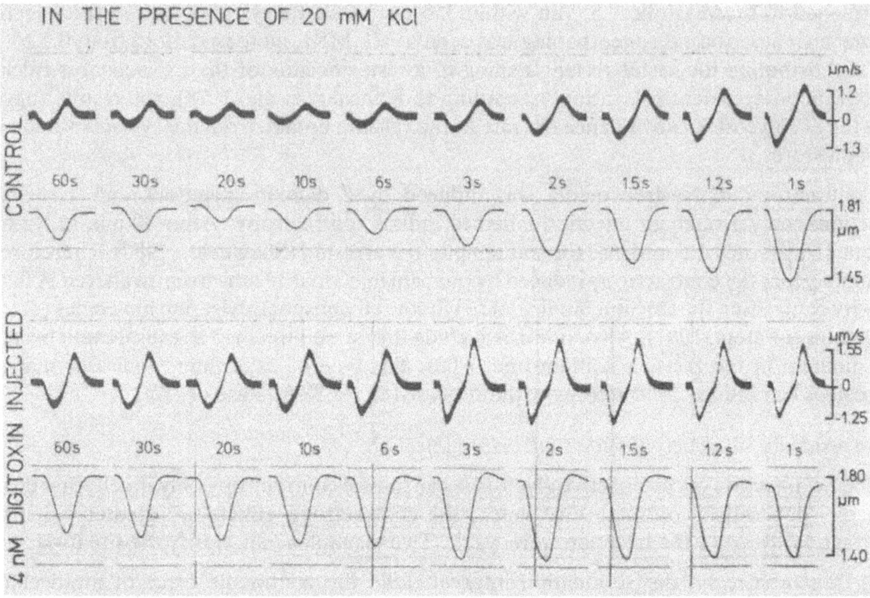

Fig. 9. Dependence of the contractropy on the stimulation interval (varied between 60 s and 1 s). Stimulation with long intervals at the beginning of the experiments. The recordings were taken, when the contractions at a given stimulation interval had reached a steady state. A: contracions and their derivatives before and 5–13 min after injection of 4 nM digitoxin.

frequency of stimulation is increased (positive Herztreppe). After the injection of 4 nM digitoxin, the dependency of ES, MRS, and MRL on the interval length is strongly attenuated (compare the curves in Fig. 9B). This means that the i.c. digitoxin increased the contractions at 10 sec long intervals about 3fold, whereas the contractions evoked at 1 Hz stimulation increased by only 1.3fold. At intervals shorter than 0.8 sec, no contractropy could be demonstrated. Thus, the contractility that was already enhanced by the higher rate of stimulation, became insensitive to the i.c. glycoside. Similar effects are known for the inotropic effects of e.c. applied glycosides (Koch-Weser & Blinks, 1962). They have been attributed to the filling of stores that release activator calcium, that is, when these stores were already filled by the "Treppe" mechanism, the glycosides can not fill them further.

b) Isolated bovine ventricular cells stimulated at 0.1 Hz respond to a doubling in $[Ca]_o$ (1.8 to 3.6 mM) with a nearly 2fold increase in ES, MRS, and MRL (Isenberg, unpublished). The curves relating ES, MRS, and MRL to the stimulation interval become flat suggesting that the i.c. calcium stores are filled to a stable level. At 3.6 mM $[Ca]_o$, i.c. injection of 2–5 nM digoxin did not increase the ES (factor less than 1.2) in 4 out of 6 cells. In the 2 other cells, ES increased 1.4 and 1.6fold. On average, elevated $[Ca]_o$ significantly inhibits the contractropy of i.c. glycosides. Such a result confirms the idea that both elevated $[Ca]_o$ and i.c. glycosides enhance the contractility via the same mechanism which is probably the loading of the SR.

Discussion

Usually, we understand "contractility" in terms of force development as measured under isometric conditions. In this paper, the contractility was evaluated by the isotonic shortening

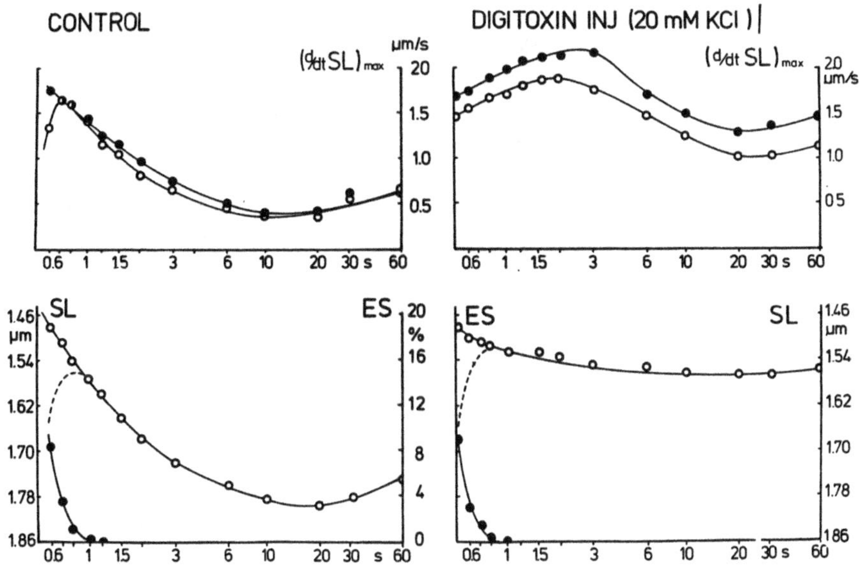

(Fig. 9 continued) B: evaluation of the data from A. Left: before, right: after injection. Bottom: amplitude of shortening (circles), incomplete diastolic relengthening (dots), and extent of shortening (broken line). Top: non-normalized rates of shortening (circles) and relengthening (dots).

of the unloaded cell. Both force development and shortening result from the transient increase in activator $[Ca]_i$. Whereas the pCa_i-force relationship is well defined (ct. ref. Fabiato, 1983), the dependence of the unloaded shortening on pCa_i is uncertain. For a better understanding, I would like to connect the events of shortening and force development with the following model: when the sarcomeres shorten, they work against an internal load distorting the myofilament lattice and bending the myosin filaments when the SL shortens below 1.65 µM. As in a spring, the internal load increases with the extent of shortening. This explains the fall of the rate of shortening with smaller SL (Isenberg, 1982). The internal load connects the parameters ES and MRS with that of the force development. It has been postulated that ES, MRS and force follow a similar dependence on pCa_i (see also DeClerck et al. 1977, 1981). The similar dependence on activator calcium is supported by comparing the interval dependence of ES and MRS (Fig. 9), which both strongly resemble the interval dependence of the isometric force (Koch-Weser & Blinks, 1962). It is extrapolated that “contractropy“ (defined here as increase in ES and MRS) and inotropy (increase in force) result from the same event, the transient increase in activator $[Ca]_i$.

As an additional parameter of the “contractropy”, the MRL was introduced. According to Brutsaert et al. (1978), the relaxation should be split into a first “activation dependent” part representing the re-normalization of activator $[Ca]_i$ and the break down of crossbridges, and a second “load dependent” part where the restoring force renormalizes the SL. In the spring model, the restoring force comes from the kinetic energy stored in the internal load (bending of the myosin filaments, see also Fabiato & Fabiato, 1976). A contraction of greater ES stores more kinetic energy in the “spring” which re-lengthens the sarcomeres faster. This load dependent relaxation superimposes upon the “activation dependent part”, i.e. it can start only when renormalization of activator calcium provides the break down of the cross bridges. Thus, a faster fall in $[Ca]_i$ (e.g. due to a faster rate of calcium uptake into the SR) should enhance the MRL. Since the cardiac glycosides do not act on the level of the contractile proteins (Katz, 1966) it seems to be clear that they enhance the contractility by increasing the amount of activator calcium (Allen & Blinks, 1978, Blinks et al., 1982).

The results of this paper show that i.c. nanomolar concentrations of cardioactive glycosides enhance the contractility; this "contractropy" was characterized by a greater extent of shortening (ES), by a faster maximal rate of shortening (MRS), and a faster maximal rate of re-lengthening (MRL). The contractropy due to i.c. injected glycosides did not necessarily require $[Na]_i$-load, inhibition of the Na,K-ATPase or the interaction with its extracellular receptor. The contractropy necessarily required the presence of one of the glycosides ouabain, digoxin or digitoxin in the injectans. The contractropy was "specific" for the glycosides since injections of adrenaline could not mimic their effect. Whether or not the contractropy can be induced by injecting "unspecific" steroids has not yet been tested. Comparing the i.c. injected ouabain, digoxin, digitoxin and albumin-conjugated digoxin, they augmented the ES within the same half time of 70 sec and by a similar degree. This result suggests that the drugs bind to a "site" facing the i.c. water without diffusional barriers. It further suggests that the drugs bind quickly, otherwise the accumulation of the (lipophilic) digitoxin in the lipids would have reduced the effective i.c. concentration.

The contractropy induced by either i.c. injected or e.c. applied glycosides was similar in many respects, and one likes to link both of them to a common underlying mechanism. One could see the "link" in a common final step that is triggered either by an e.c. or by an i.c. pathway. One could also postulate that the e.c. glycoside has to internalize before it can induce inotropy. Though the present results favour the latter point of view, they do not rule out the first one:

Since albumin-conjugated digoxin induces contractropy from the i.c.s. but not from the e.c.s., one could interpret this as meaning that the large molecule cannot internalize and therefore not act, but, in the classical interpretation the albumin residue hinders the digoxin binding to the e.c. receptor (Smith et al., 1972). Comparing the effects of e.c. applied ouabain, digoxin, digitoxin, these develop with different delays suggesting that the more lipophilic digitoxin appears in the i.c.s. more rapidly than the ouabain. But in the steady state, inotropy resulting from internalization related to lipophilicity should be 10fold greater (e.c. digitoxin compared with e.c. ouabain) and it is similar (similar concentrations and long time exposure give for digitoxin a 10fold higher tissue to medium radioactivity than for ouabain, Lüllmann et al., 1975). Internalization via the lipid bilayer also can not explain that the effects of e.c. glycosides are inhibited by high $[K]_o$ or low $[Na]_o$. Perhaps, the lipophilic glycosides accumulate in a compartment (the lipids) which is not relevant for contractropy. Thus, one speculates that glycosides internalize via a carrier mediated transport (Dutta et al., 1968; Fricke et al., 1969; Park & Vincenzi, 1975; Fricke, 1978). (A ouabain carrier has been described in hepatocytes by e.g. Stacey & Klaasen, 1979; Schwenk et al., 1981.)

What might be the underlying mechanism that enhances the activator calcium? According to the literature, one may distinguish mechanisms that fill the i.c. stores to a greater extent and those that facilitate the release (cf. rev. Klaus & Lee, 1969; Lee & Klaus, 1971). Both of them should imply an intact sarcolemmal membrane since application of glycosides to the i.c.s. of preparations with skinned membranes evoked neither inotropy nor increases in the activator calcium (Fabiato & Fabiato, 1973, Nayler, 1973).

1. The i.c. glycosides act by inhibiting the Ca-efflux, the extra calcium filling the SR. (As long as the SR is not overcharged, the time to peak and the maximum rate of relengthening do not necessarily have to increase.) Regarding the underlying processes, the involvement of the Na-Ca exchange mechanism (cf. ref. Reuter, 1983) is unlikely because contractropy was also induced in Na-free media (p. 11). The transsarcolemmal Ca-ATPase (cf. ref. Caroni &

Carafoli, 1981) is sensitive to glycosides, however, the effects were seen only in perfused hearts where the glycosides could bind to the e.c. Na,K-ATPase receptor and not in sarcolemmal inside out vesicles (Lüllmann et al., 1982; Preuner, 1983).

2. The sarcoplasmic Ca-ATPase (cf. ref. Hasselbach, 1982) is stimulated by glycosides. Such a mechanism could easily account for both the greater ES and the faster MRL (see esp. Fig. 8). It could also explain the requirement of a non-potentiated state (e.g. $[Ca]_o < 3.6$ mM, stimulation frequencies <1 Hz). Such a "ceiling off" (Koch-Weser & Blinks, 1962, 1963) suggests that additional filling of stores already loaded to their optimum is either not possible or uneffective. Since no consistent effect on the SR calcium uptake of microsomes has been reported (Lee & Klaus, 1971), this could mean that the hypothetical mechanisms are destroyed when the SR loses its contact with the sarcolemma, that the glycosides act via a non-membrane bound mediator, or that the SR calcium pump is not the target of the i.c. glycosides.

3. The i.c. glycosides could stimulate the Ca-influx. Stimulation of a transsarcolemmal Ca-K exchange (Morad & Greenspan, 1973) would explain both $[Ca]_i$-load and abbreviation of the action potential (Fig. 8), but direct evidence for such a mechanisms as yet missing. An increase in the slow inward calcium current has been described recently for e.c. applied glycosides (Marban & Tsien, 1982). Provided that i.c. glycosides act the same, they would enhance the calcium entry during the plateau of the action potential.

4. The i.c. glycosides could stimulate the calcium release from i.c. stores. Regarding the phospholipids of the sarcolemma as the "store", it was suggested that binding of glycosides to the e.c. receptor alters the conformation of the Na,K-ATPase which leads to a change in the calcium affinity of negatively charged groups (Besch & Schwartz, 1970; Lüllmann & Peters, 1976). Whether or not such an effect can be induced by i.c. glycosides has not yet been tested.

5. The i.c. glycosides could facilitate the calcium release from the SR. In mechanically skinned heart fibres, the calcium induced calcium release was not enhanced by ouabain (Fabiato & Fabiato, 1973). In microsomes from heart SR, exposure to 1 μM ouabain for 1 min stimulated the release induced by depolarization by 4fold but not the release induced by caffeine (Fujino et al., 1979). Thus, depolarization induced calcium release from the SR seems to be a mechanism which facilitated by i.c. glycosides could provide the cell with more activator calcium and thereby enhance its contractility.

References

Allen DG, Blinks JR (1978) Calcium transients in aequorin injected frog cardiac muscle. Nature (London) 273:509–513

Besch HR, Schwartz A (1970) On a mechanism of action of digitalis. J. mol. cell. Cardiol. 1:195–199

Blinks JR, Wier G, Morgan JP, Hess P Regulation of intracellular $[Ca^{2+}]$ by cardiotonic drugs. In: Advances in Pharmacology and Therapeutics II, vol 3. ed Yoshida J, Hagiwara Y, Ebashi S (Pergamon Press Oxford)

Brutsaert OL, Claes VA, DeClerck NM (1978) Relaxation of mammalian single cardiac cells after pretreatment with the detergent Brij-58. J Physiol (Lond.) 283:481–491

Caroni P, Carafoli E (1981) An ATP-dependent Ca^{2+}-pumping ATPase of heart sarcolemma. J Biol Chem 256:3263–3270

DeClerck NM, Claes VA, Brutsaert DL (1977) Force velocity relations of single cardiac muscle cells. J Gen Physiol 69:221–241

DeClerck NM, Claes VA, Ocken ER, Brutsaert DL (1981) Sarcomere distribution patterns in single cardiac cells. Biophys J 35:237–242

Dreyer F, Peper K (1974) Iontophoretic application of acetylcholine: advantage of high resistance micropipettes in connection with an electronic current pump. Pflügers Arch 348:253–272

Dutta S, Marks BH (1972) Species and ionic influeces on the accumulation of digitalis glycosides by isolated perfused hearts. Br J Pharmacol 46:401–408

Dutta S, Goswam S, Datta DK, Lindower JA, Marks BH (1968) The uptake and binding of six radiolabeled cardiac glydosides by guinea pig hearts and by isolated sarcoplasmic reticulum. J Pharmacol Exp Ther 164:10–21

Endo, M (1977) Calcium release from the sarcoplasmic reticulum. Physiol Rev 57:71–108

Fabiato A, Fabiato F (1973) Activation of skinned cardiac cells. Subcellular effects of cardioactive drugs. Europ J Cardiology 1:143–155

Fabiato A, Fabiato F (1976) Dependence of calcium release, tension generation and restoring forces on sarcomere length in skinned cardiac cells. Europ J Cardiology 4:13–27

Fabiato A (1983) Calcium-induced release of calcium from the cardiac sarcoplasmic reticulum. Am J Physiol 245:C1–C14

Fricke U (1978) Myocardial activity of inhibitors of the Na-K-ATPase: difference in the mode of action and subcellular pattern of N-ethylamide and ouabain. Naunyn-Schmiedeberg's Arch Pharmacol 303:197–204

Fricke U, Klaus W (1977) Evidence for two different Na-dependent [3H]-ouabain binding sites of a Na-K-ATPase of guinea-pig hearts. Br J Pharmac 61:423–428

Fricke U, Klaus W (1971) Comparative studies of the influence of various K-concentrations on the action of k-strophanthidin, digitoxin and strophanthidin-3-bromoacetate on papillary muscle and on membrane ATPase of guinea pig hearts. European J Pharmocol 15:1–7

Fricke U, Klaus W (1978) Sodium-dependent cardiac glycoside binding: experimental evidence and hypothesis. Br J Pharmacol 62:255–257

Fujino S, Igarashi T, Hoshi K (1979) Ouabain potentiation of Ca release from fragmented cardiac sarcoplasmic reticulum. Japan J Pharmacol 29:839–845

Greenspan AM, Morad M (1975) Electromechanical studies on the inotropic effects of acetylstrophanthidin in ventricular muscle. J Physiol 253:357–384

Hasselbach W (1978) The reversibility of the sarcoplasmic calcium pump. Biochim Biophys Acta 515:25–53

Hess P, Müller P (1982) Extracellular versus intracellular digoxin action on bovine myocardium, using a digoxin antibody and intracellular glycoside application. J Physiol (Lond.) 322:197–210

Isenberg G (1977) Cardiac Purkinje fibers. Resting, action, and pacemaker potential under the influence of $[Ca]_i$ as modified by intracellular injection techniques. Pflügers Arch 371:51–59

Isenberg G (1979) Risk and advantages of using strongly beveled microelectrodes for electrophysiological studies in cardiac Purkinje fibers. Pflügers Arch 380:91–98

Isenberg G (1982) Ca entry and contraction as studied in isolated bovine ventricular myocytes. Z Naturforsch 37c:502–512

Isenberg G, Klöckner U (1982) Calcium tolerant ventricular myocytes prepared by preincubation in a "KB medium". Pflügers Arch 395:6–18

Katz AM (1971) Absence of effects of cardiac glycosides on cardiac myosin and a Ca^{2+}-sensitive reconstituted cardiac actomyosin. J Pharmacol Exp Ther 154:558–565

Klaus W, Fricke U (1978) Electrolyte-dependence of cardiac glycoside actions at the cellular and subcellular level. In: Recent Advances in Studies on Cardiac Structure and Metabolism Vol 11, 393–399. Eds Kobayashi T, Sano T, Dhalla NS. University Park Press

Klaus W, Lee KS (1969) Influence of cardiac glycosides on calcium binding in muscle subcellular components. J Pharmacol Exp Ther 166:68–76

Koch-Weser J, Blinks JR (1962) Analysis of the relation of the positive inotropic action of cardiac glycosides to the frequency of contraction of heart muscle. J Pharmacol Exp Ther 136:305–317

Koch-Weser J, Blinks JR (1963) The influence of the interval between beats on myocardial contractility. Pharmacol Rev 15:601–652

Lee KS, Klaus W (1971) The subcellular basis for the mechanism of inotropic action of cardiac glycosides. Pharmacol Rev 23:193–261

Lüllmann H, Peters T (1981) Influence of cardiac glycosides on cell membrane. In: Greeff K (ed) Handbook of experimental Pharmacology, Vol 56/I, p 395–406 (Springer Berlin–Heidelberg)

Lüllmann H, Peters T, Preuner J (1982) Mechanism of the action of digitalis glycosides in the light of new experimental observations. Europ Heart J 3B:45–51

Lüllmann H, Peters T, Ravens U (1975) Studies on the kinetics of [^{3}H]-ouabain uptake and exchange in the isolated papillary muscle of the guinea pig. Br J Pharmac 53:99–107

Marban E, Tsien RW (1982) Enhancement of calcium current during digitalis inotropy in mammalian heart: positive feed-back regulation by intracellular calcium? J Physiol 329:589–614
Nayler WG (1973) Effect of inotropic agents on canine trabecular muscle rendered highly permeable to calcium. Am J Physiol 225:918–924
Park MK, Vicenzi FF (1975) Rate of onset of cardiotonic steroid-induced inotropism: influence of temperature and beat interval. J Pharmacol Exp Ther 195:140–150
Page E (1978) Quantitative ultrastructural analysis in cardiac membrane physiology. Am J Physiol 235:C147–C158
Preuner J (1983) Ouabain induced inhibition of the cardiac sarolemmal Ca-pump and (Ca^{2+},Mg^{2+}) transport ATPase accompanied by a stimulation of the Mg^{2+}-ATPase activity. Naunyn-Schmiedeberg's Arch Pharmacol 322:R27
Prindle KH, Skelton CL, Epstein SE (1971) Influence of extracellular potassium concentration on myocardial uptake and inotropic effect of tritiated digoxin. Circ Res 28:337–345
Reiter M (1962) Die Entstehung von "Nachkontraktionen" im Herzmuskel unter Einwirkung von Calcium und von Digitalisglycosiden in Abhängigkeit von der Reizfrequenz. Naunyn-Schmiedeberg's Arch Pharmacol 242:487–507
Reuter H (1982) Na-Ca countertransport in cardiac muscle. In: Membranes and Transport, Vol 1 Ed by A Martonosi, Plenum Press, New York and London
Schwenk M, Wiedmann T, Remmer H (1981) Uptake, accumulation and release of ouabain by isolated rat hepatocytes. Naunyn-Schmiedeberg's Arch Pharmacol 316:340–344
Sheu S-S, Korth M, Lathrop DA, Fozzard HA (1980) Intra- and extracellular K^+ and Na^+ activities and resting membrane potential in sheep cardiac Purkinje strands. Circ Res 47:692–700
Smith TW, Curd JG, Haber E (1971) Rapid reversal of digoxin toxicity by Fab fragments from purified digoxin specific antibody. Circulation 44:11–41
Smith TW, Haber E (1972) Digitalis. Little Brown & Comp., (Boston)
Smith TW, Wagner H, Markis JE (1972) Studies on the localization of the cardiac glycoside receptor. J Clin Invest 51:1777–1789
Stacey NH, Klaassen CD (1979) Uptake of ouabain by isolated hepatocytes from livers of developing rats. J Pharmacol Exp Ther 211:360–363
Wasserstrom JA, Schwartz DJ, Fozzard HA (1983) Relation between intracellular sodium and twitch tension in sheep cardiac Purkinje strands exposed to cardiac glycosides. Circ Res, 52:697–705
Weingart R (1974) The permeability to tetraethylammonium ions of the surface membrane and the intercalated disks of sheep and calf myocardium. J Physiol (Lond) 240:741–762

Author's address:

Dr. G. Isenberg, II. Physiologisches Institut der Universität des Saarlandes, D 6650 Homburg/Saar

The electrogenic Na-K pump current and actions of the cardiac glycosides

D. Noble

University Laboratory of Physiology, Oxford (England)

Key words: Purkinje fibres, cardiac glycosides, potassium, membrane current, $(Na^{+}+K^{+})$-ATPase

Introduction

In 1974, Isenberg and Trautwein measured an outward current in sheep cardiac Purkinje fibres that was nearly independent of membrane potential and which they attributed to current generated by the Na-K exchange pump. Their method involved measuring the ionic current-voltage relation before and immediately after application of a fast-acting and reversible cardiac glycoside, dihydro-ouabain. I will refer to current generated by the Na-K pump as i_p.

Isenberg & Trautwein's method however rarely measures i_p alone. In the majority of experiments on sheep Purkinje fibres, there are also substantial variations in current attributable to changes in the extracellular [K] concentration. These were investigated by Cohen, Daut & Noble (1976) who found that, particularly at fairly negative potentials where the current carried by the inward rectifier, i_{Kl}, is substantial, changes in i_K due to changes in the cleft [K] concentration can easily dominate the net current change. The total current change, Δi, is then composed of two elements:

$$\Delta i = i_p + \Delta i_{Kl} \quad (1)$$

This was not the only complexity noted by Cohen et al. They also found that, at glycoside concentrations in the therapeutic range (10^{-9} to 10^{-8}M), the potassium ionic concentration gradient, as estimated using the second term in equation (1), changes in the *opposite* direction to that expected for pump inhibition.

In this paper I shall briefly review the work on i_p since Isenberg & Trautwein's paper. I shall then discuss the actions of high and low concentrations of cardiac glycosides.

Measurement of i_p

Clearly, to measure i_p accurately, it is important to seek conditions in which changes due to i_{Kl} (or any other currents that may change when $[K]_o$, $[Na]_i$ or $[Ca]_i$ change) are minimised. Three possible techniques are now available. Eisner & Lederer (1980) and Eisner, Lederer & Vaughan-Jones (1982) used Rb^+ as a substitute for K^+. The justification for this approach is that the Rb^+ current does not show the same degree of inward-going rectification as does K^+ (i.e. the inward current carried through the i_{Kl} channels is very small). This largely eliminates the second term in equation (1). Yet, it is well known that Rb^+ is not only an activator of the Na-K pump, but that it is equally effective as K^+. The second approach is to use Purkinje fibre preparations that have much larger extracellular spaces so minimising the changes due to variations in the cleft K^+ concentration $[K]_c$. This is the approach used by Gadsby (1980) who used canine Purkinje fibres which have a much larger extracellular space (Eisenberg & Cohen, 1983). Daut & Rüdel (1982) have described measurements of i_p in ventricular tissue that may be less contaminated by variations in $[K]_c$ than in sheep Purkinje fibres. The third possibility is to use single cells with no restricted extracellular space. Shibata, Momose & Giles (1983) have recently reported measurements of i_p in isolated single frog atrial cells.

Although cardiac glycosides have been used to induce variations in i_p in this work, by far the more useful technique has been to use K^+-free solutions to inhibit the pump. The protocol is now fairly well established. The cells are first exposed to K^+-free solution for a period, about 10 minutes, sufficient to allow a substantial rise in intracellular sodium, $[Na]_i$, to occur. Typically, $[Na]_i$ is allowed to rise from its resting level near 8 mM to about 20 mM in this period of time (see Ellis, 1977; Deitmer & Ellis, 1978; Eisner, Lederer & Vaughan-Jones, 1981). The cells are then returned to solutions containing various concentrations of the external activator cation (K^+ or Rb^+). The raised $[Na]_i$ then stimulates the activity of the Na-K exchange pump

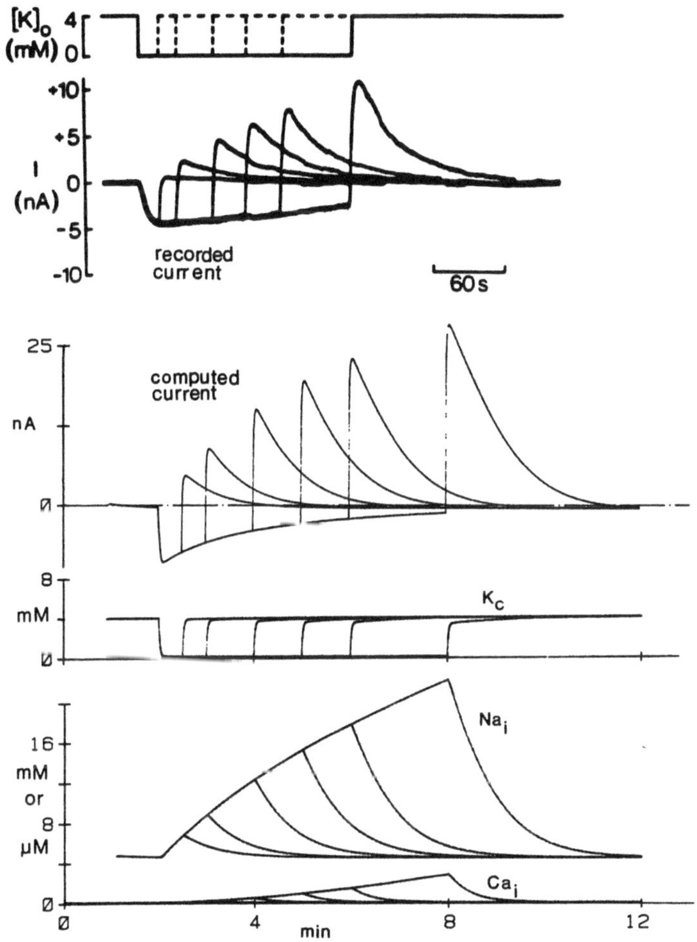

Fig. 1. Top: Membrane current changes recorded during reactivation of the Na^+/K^+ pump following various periods of exposure to K^+-free solution in a canine Purkinje fibre (Gadsby 1980).
Bottom: Computed membrane currents and variations in $[K]_c$, $[Na]_i$ and $[Ca]_i$ using a similar protocol on a mathematical model of Purkinje fibre electrical activity (DiFrancesco & Noble, 1982, 1984).

thus producing an outward current, i_p, that decays as $[Na]_i$ returns towards its resting level. The magnitude of i_p recorded in this way can be varied either by varying the concentration of activator cation or by varying the duration of K^+-free superfusion (thus varying the increase in $[Na]_i$). Figure 1A shows an example of the latter approach from an experiment described by Gadsby (1980). On return to K^+-containing solution there is an outward current that decays exponentially with a time constant of about 2 minutes, which is about the time constant of the change in $[Na]_i$.

This approach has been very valuable in characterising the Na-K pump in cardiac cells. Gadsby's own work shows that $[K]_o$ activates the pump in the way expected, with half-activation occurring at about 1 mM. By also measuring $[Na]_i$, Eisner et al. were also able to assess the dependence on $[Na]_i$, which is linear over the range investigated (up to about 25 mM). Interestingly, Eisner, Lederer & Vaughan-Jones obtain a considerably higher value for the K_m for activation by external K^+ than that obtained by Gadsby. It is possible that this is due to effects of the restricted extracellular space in sheep preparations rather than to a genuine difference in K_m for activation.

The data obtained from these experiments has recently been incorporated into a model of electrical activity in Purkinje fibres (DiFrancesco & Noble, 1982, 1984) and a simulation of Gadsby's experiment using the model equations is shown in figure 1B. There is fairly good correspondence between the behaviour of the model and the experimental results, including the fact that, during the exposure to K^+-free solution, there is a small upward creep in the current record. In the model, this is due to residual activation of i_p by cleft $[K]_c$ (which, of course, never falls to zero even in a nominally K^+-free solution). This residual i_p then increases as $[Na]_i$ increases.

Eisner, Lederer & Vaughan-Jones (1981, 1983a, b) also measured tension during experiments of this kind and have produced some excellent correlations between the level of $[Na]_i$ and the magnitude of the twitch and tonic tensions. This work gives a clear quantitative basis to the so-called Na-lag theory of tension increase during sodium pump inhibition. It is worth noting, in particular, that the relation between tension and $[Na]_i$ is very steep. Fairly small changes (e.g. only 1 mM) in $[Na]_i$ can correlate with large changes in force.

Daut & Rüdel (1982) have used dihydro-ouabain to inhibit the pump in their experiments on ventricular muscle. This approach has permitted them to describe accurately the changes in action potential duration that occur during pump inhibition and associated tension changes. These are usually biphasic. Initially the changes that occur are consistent with a removal of i_p, which would be a repolarizing current, so leading to action potential prolongation. Later, the action potential shortens. This may be due to effects of consequent changes in $[Ca]_i$ on currents other than i_p.

Gadsby & Cranefield (1982) have described another way of demonstrating that i_p contributes to the repolarizing current during the action potential. This is to measure the shortening of the action potential when i_p is transiently increased during experiments of the kind shown in figure 1. This effect is also well reproduced by the DiFrancesco-Noble (1984) model.

What determines the normal level of i_p?

The fact that external [K] concentrations over the range 0–6 mM have a large effect on i_p might lead one to expect large variations in i_p during natural variations in $[K]_o$. Daut (1983) has measured i_p in guinea-pig ventricular muscle when $[K]_o$ is varied between 2 and 4.5 mM. He found no significant variation in i_p. As he argues in his paper, this result is not surprising. When one solves the appropriate steady-state equations one finds that the *steady state* magnitude of i_p should depend on the passive sodium influx and there is no reason to expect this to vary with $[K]_o$ (cf Cohen, Daut & Noble, 1976; Gadsby, 1980). The explanation of the relatively constant value of i_p is that variations in $[Na]_i$ occur that bring the pump activity, and hence i_p, back to the steady state value within a minute or two following a perturbation. Another way of putting this point is to say that there is sufficient spare capacity in the pump mechanism for changes in $[Na]_i$ to readily bring the pump towards a constant resting value. A corollary of this high »gain« shown by the pump is that it will require a fairly substantial amount of pump inhibition to produce a significant change in resting steady state pump activity. Morever, factors that may stimulate the pump (see below) would be expected to produce only transient increases in pump activity.

An important consequence of this relatively constant level of the resting i_p is that the relation between cardiac glycoside concentration and i_p cannot be used to measure glycoside binding since a substantial degree of binding (and of pump inhibition) may occur with little or no change in i_p. This effect has been reproduced quantitatively by Hart, Noble & Shimoni (1983) using the DiFrancesco-Noble (1982, 1984) equations.

Influence of high and low concentrations of cardiac glycosides

There is no doubt that relatively high ($>5 \times 10^{-7}$ M) concentrations of cardiac glycosides reduce the pump current, i_p, either transiently (during moderate inhibition) or permanently (during strong inhibition). The more controversial question is what happens at much lower concentrations towards and in the therapeutic range. Cohen, Daut & Noble (1976) found that, at low concentrations, the current changes (both in i_p and in correlated changes in i_{K1}) are those expected from *stimulation* rather than from inhibition of the Na-K pump. Hart, Noble & Shimoni (1983) have recently re-investigated the situation in Purkinje fibres, combining measurements of tension with recordings of the currents under voltage clamp conditions. Figure 2 summarizes their results. At a ouabain concentration of 5×10^{-8} M two-thirds of the preparations showed the "stimulatory" effect. Near 10^{-7} M, "stimulatory" and "inhibitory" effects occur almost equally. At 5×10^{-7} M, the inhibitory effect clearly dominates.

The stimulatory change in current (an outward current increase) is usually only transient, as expected from the argument presented in the previous section. Gadsby (1983) has also sometimes observed the small outward current increase at low concentrations and Ellis (1977) and Deitmer & Ellis (1978) have recorded a very small fall in intracellular sodium at low glycoside concentrations.

The effect has now been seen by different workers and with different techniques. It is not likely therefore to be an artefact. What is its significance?

In 1980 (Noble 1980) I reviewed this effect extensively in relation to the many other reports that low concentrations of cardiac glycosides may stimulate the Na-K exchange pump and suggested both that this effect was related to the other observations suggesting stimulation of the pump or of isolated Na-K ATPase and that there might be advantages in describing the effect as a form of "disinhibition".

The obvious alternative explanation is that the effect is not a direct action of cardiac glycosides on the cardiac cell membrane but rather an indirect effect due, for example, to change in activity of nerve endings in the preparation. Hougen & Smith (1980) have argued from their observations showing that the "stimulatory" effect is absent in reserpinised preparations that the effect may be due to release of catecholamines from nerve endings. This effect may well occur. But it is important to note that it cannot explain the results obtained by Hart, Noble & Shimoni (1983). There are two reasons for this:

1. In about half the preparations showing the "stimulatory" effect, there is a *negative* inotropic response, which is opposite to that expected from the well-known positive inotropic action of catecholamines. This effect is though *precisely* that expected from the pump-lag

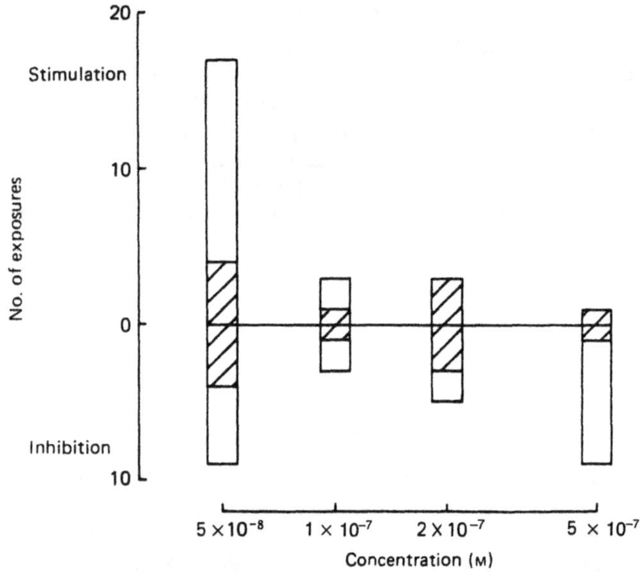

Fig. 2. Effects of different concentrations of strophanthidin and ouabain on the presumed direction of change of net pump activity in 5.4 mM $[K]_o$ and 2 mM $[Ca]_o$. The white areas show results giving only stimulation or only inhibition. Some experiments gave transient stimulation before inhibition. These are shown as the hatched areas. For further details, see Hart et al. (1983).

hypothesis. A small fall in $[Na]_i$ due to stimulation of the pump would reduce $[Ca]_i$ and so produce a negative inotropic response.

2. In the relevant range of potentials, the electrical effect of catecholamines has already been measured in cardiac Purkinje fibres. The result is a net *inward* current shift (as indeed it must be if catecholamines are to accelerate the pacemaker potential) which is opposite to that found in Hart et al's (15) experiments.

The negative inotropic effect associated with the "stimulatory" effect in about half the experiments is, I think, very important. We were not the first to describe this effect (see (15) for references) but it tends to be neglected partly because it is often (though not always – see (15) figure 8) very small and partly because the much more accepted action is the well-known and much larger positive inotropic response.

It is important, though, to note that in some experiments the "stimulatory" effect on membrane current *is* nevertheless associated with a net positive inotropic effect. When this effect occurs, it is usually possible to distinguish it from the larger positive inotropic effect associated with pump inhibition. Like the effect on membrane current, it is often transient. In one particularly illustrative experiment (see Figure 3) we were able to record a small transient positive inotropic response while the membrane current was shifting in the outward direction during the first 5 minutes of exposure to strophanthidin, while recording a slower and much larger positive inotropic effect during the later inward shift in membrane current. In this case, the first tension change reversed before the second one began.

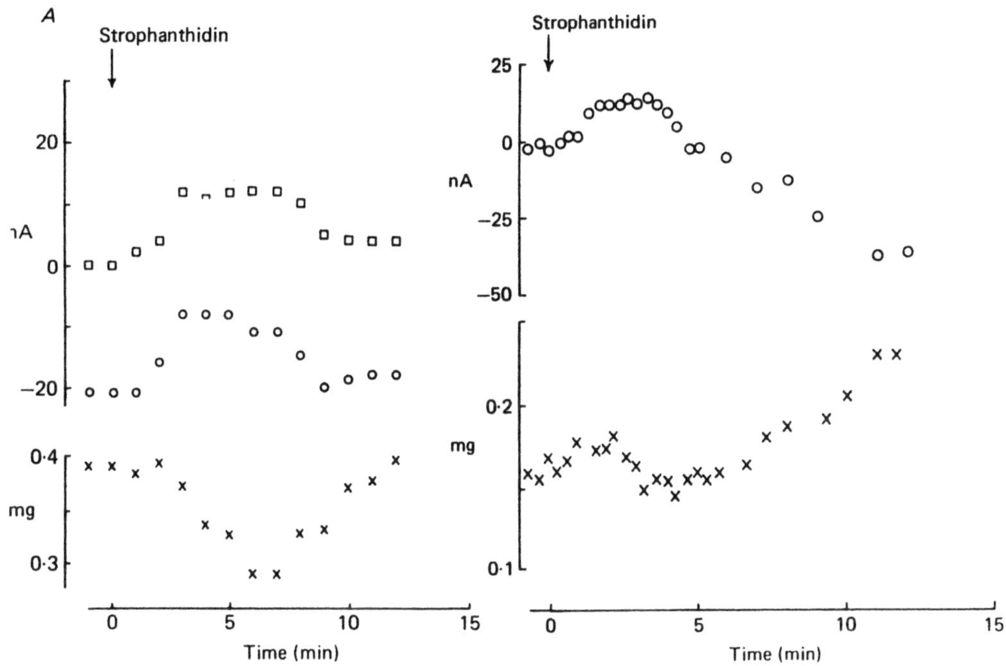

Fig. 3. Results of two experiments in which the Purkinje fibre was exposed to 5×10^{-8} M strophanthidin. In both cases transient outward current shifts were recorded. The preparation on the left showed only this effect which was accompanied by a substantial *negative* inotropic effect. The fibre on the right showed a transient outward shift before a permanent inward shift (this is an example of a "hatched" case in Figure 2). A small *positive* inotropic effect accompanied the outward current shift. A larger and much slower positive inotropic effect accompanied the inward shift. (From Hart et al., 1983).

Conclusions

The sodium pump current, i_p, is now sufficiently well characterised in cardiac muscle to be incorporated into electrical models of excitation and for a sufficient explanation of the contribution of i_p to the resting and action potential to be obtained.

Under steady state conditions, i_p will be relatively constant despite fairly wide variations in $[K]_o$. The steady state level of activity may also be nearly constant at therapeutic levels of cardiac glycosides since any stimulatory or inhibitory effects of non-toxic concentrations may well be too small to overcome the natural "gain" of the pump.

There is no doubt that high concentrations of cardiac glycosides reduce i_p, but there is also evidence that very low concentrations may transiently increase i_p. The significance of this effect in relation to the therapeutic actions of cardiac glycosides, and in relation to the question of more than one binding site remains unclear.

Acknowledgements

The work in my own laboratory is supported by the Medical Research Council and by the British Heart Foundation.

References

1. Cohen I, Daut J, Noble D (1976) An analysis of the actions of low concentrations of ouabain on membrane currents in Purkinje fibres. J Physiol 260:75–103
2. Daut J (1983) Inhibition of the sodium pump in guinea-pig ventricular muscle by dihydro-ouabain: effects of external potassium and sodium. J Physiol 339:643–662
3. Daut J, Rüdel R (1982) The electrogenic sodium pump in guinea-pig ventricular muscle: inhibition of pump current by cardiac glycosides. J Physiol 330:243–264
4. Deitmer JW, Ellis D (1978) The intracellular sodium activity of cardiac Purkinje fibres during inhibition and re-activation of the Na-K pump. J Physiol 284:241–259
5. DiFrancesco D, Noble D (1982) Implications of the re-interpretation of i_{K2} for the modelling of the electrical activity of pacemaker tissues in the heart. In: Cardiac Rate and Rhythm Bouman LN, Jongsma HB Ed pp 93–128 (Martinus Nijhoff The Hague)
6. DiFrancesco D, Noble D (1984) A model of cardiac electrical activity incorporating ionic pumps and concentration changes. Phil. Trans. Roy. Soc. (in press).
7. Eisenberg BR, Cohen IS (1983) The ultrastructure of the cardiac Purkinje strand in the dog: a morphometric analysis. Proc. Roy. Soc. B217:191–213
8. Eisner DA, Lederer WJ (1980) Characterisation of the sodium pump in cardiac Purkinje fibres. J Physiol 303:441–474
9. Eisner DA, Lederer WJ, Vaughan-Jones RD (1981) The dependence of sodium pumping and tension on intracellular sodium activity in voltage-clamped sheep Purkinje fibres. J Physiol 317:163–187
10. Eisner DA, Lederer WJ, Vaughan-Jones RD (1983a) The control of tonic tension by membrane potential and intracellular sodium activity in the sheep cardiac Purkinje fibre. J Physiol 335:723–743
11. Eisner DA, Lederer WJ, Vaughan-Jones RD (1983b) The relationship between twitch tension and intracellular sodium activity in sheep cardiac Purkinje fibres. J Physiol 341:28–29P
12. Ellis D (1977) The effects of external cations and ouabain on the intracellular sodium activity of sheep heart Purkinje fibres. J Physiol 273:211–240
13. Gadsby DC (1980) Activation of electrogenic Na^+/K^+ exchange by extracellular K^+ in canine cardiac Purkinje fibres. J gen Physiol 65:345–365
14. Gadsby DC, Cranefield PF (1982) Effects of electrogenic sodium extrusion on the membrane potential of cardiac Purkinje fibres. In: Normal and Abnormal Conduction in the Heart. Paes de Carvalho A, Hoffman BF, Lieberman M Eds pp 225–247 (Futura Publishing Company, NY Mount Kisco)
15. Hart G, Noble D, Shimoni Y (1983) The effects of low concentrations of cardiotonic steroids on membrane currents and tension in sheep Purkinje fibres. J Physiol 334:103–131
16. Hougen TJ, Smith TW (1980) Biphasic effect of cardiac glycosides on the sodium pump: role of catecholamines. Circulation 62:981–987
17. Isenberg G, Trautwein W (1974) The effect of dihydro-ouabain and lithium ions on the outward current in cardiac Purkinje fibres. Evidence for electrogenicity of transport. Pflüger's Archiv 395:41–54
18. Noble D (1980) Review: mechanism of action of therapeutic levels of cardiac glycosides. Cardiovascular Research 14:495–514
19. Shibata EF, Momose Y, Giles WR (1983) Measurement of an electrogenic Na^+/K^+ pump current in individual bullfrog atrial myocytes. Proc Int Union of Physiol Sci 15:51

Author's address:

Dr. Denis Noble, University Laboratory of Physiology, Parks Road, Oxford (England)

Effects of non-toxic doses of ouabain on sodium, potassium, calcium distribution in guinea pig papillary muscle. Electronprobe microanalysis

M. F. Wendt-Gallitelli and R. Jacob

Physiologisches Institut II der Universität Tübingen (FRG)

Summary

The mechanisms and the cellular structures which are definitely involved in the accumulation and release of calcium in heart muscle treated with cardiac glycosides are not yet known.

The distribution of sodium, potassium and calcium in small papillary muscles of the guinea pig right ventricle was examined with the aid of energy dispersive x-ray microanalysis and cryotechniques. The primary aim of the present study was twofold: firstly, to determine whether an increase in intracellular sodium concentration is detectable in muscles showing positive inotropy resulting from treatment with non-toxic doses of ouabain; and secondly, whether at the end of diastole cellular stores are detectable accumulating Ca which could be responsible for the pronounced contraction which normally would follow.

Analyses on interstitium, cell membrane, sarcomeres, Z-lines and mitochondria of 7 muscles strips treated with non-toxic doses of ouabain and frozen at the end of diastole showed the following: sodium concentration in the sarcoplasm was significantly higher than over the mitochondria; it was also higher than over the sarcoplasm of non-treated muscles frozen at the end of diastole. High calcium concentrations were also measured over the cell membrane. These calcium concentrations were higher than that detected in sarcomeres, Z-lines and mitochondria. Over the sarcomeres, the calcium concentration was higher than in experiments on non-treated muscles which were also frozen at the end of diastole. Mitochondria did not accumulate any detectable concentration of calcium. The comparison of the present results with those obtained from analysis on muscles frozen after other positive inotropic interventions indicate the following cardiac glycoside-specific effects: 1) increase in intracellular sodium concentration; 2) accumulation of high calcium mass fraction during diastole in structures connected with the cell membrane – their role in activation of contraction remains to be proved – and 3) increased calcium concentration over the sarcomeres. The results strongly support the classical hypothesis that cardiac glycosides act via inhibition of the Na-K pump. Such inhibition, involving the Na/Ca exchange, would lead to an increase in cytoplasmic calcium which, in turn, is finally responsible for the positive inotropic effect.

Key words: Ouabain; electronprobe microanalysis; calcium stores; intracellular sodium

Introduction

There is no general agreement about the way cardiac glycosides act on heart muscle. The question still remains, whether the positive inotropic effect of cardiac glycosides is a consequence of inhibition of the Na^{+}-K^{+} pump, or whether positive inotropy and inhibition of the pump are non causal-linked, independent events (2, 5, 6, 10). Besides detecting a change in Na-K distribution, a contribution to the answer to this question can be given by detecting the direct origin of the contraction activating calcium in cardiac muscles treated with ouabain, and by identifying the sites of calcium buffering during diastole.

The experiments described and discussed below are part of a study started in order to answer the following questions:

1. Is it possible, by means of electron probe microanalysis on shock frozen muscles, to detect intracellular ionic shifts, in this case an increase in intracellular Na^+ and a decrease in intracellular K^+, in preparations treated with therapeutic, but non-toxic doses of ouabain? Moreover where these ionic shifts have been demonstrated with electron probe at therapeutic doses, could they also be detected at lower doses? In the latter case there is some doubt as to whether the inhibition of the Na-K pump has any bearing on the mechanism of increased force development (2, 5, 6).

2. Is it possible, by means of the same methods, to detect structures in heart muscle showing a clear accumulation of calcium at the end of diastole; that is at a time when a stimulus would produce a pronounced contraction?

3. Where sites of calcium storage have been identified at the end of diastole, are those stores involved in activating contraction? In other words, are these stores "empty" of calcium at such an early time of the contraction-relaxation cycle, that the calcium supposed to be released from these stores into the sarcoplasm can activate contraction?

Material and methods

Free papillary muscles and trabeculae with a diameter of 200–500 μm were quickly dissected from the right ventricle of the beating heart of guinea pig, extracted from the anaesthetized animals (with Urethan). The muscle strips were mounted on the set-up used for superfusion of the strip, for recording of force development as well as for triggered rapid freezing. The composition of the bath solution was, in mmol/l: NaCl 130, KCl 4.9, $CaCl_2$ 1.1, $MgCl_2$ 1.2, Glucose 24, $NaHCO_3$ 20, Na_2HPO_4 0.85 (pH 7.3 and 32 °C). The muscles in the bath were stimulated with a frequency of 1 Hz. The muscles were allowed to beat for several minutes under isotonic conditions, and were then gradually stretched with a micromanipulator to the length of maximal developed tension. They were then allowed to work in steady state at this length under near isometric conditions for ca. 1½ hour. Prior to having started with ouabain treatment, paired pulse stimulation was applied to the strips. Muscles which showed no signs of damage during this inotropic intervention were then selected for experiment. The stimulation was returned to single pulses at 1 Hz and force decreased to the original level of steady state at optimal length. The superfusion was then started with a solution containing $2 \cdot 10^{-7}$ mol ouabain (Merck). Once the full positive inotropic effect was reached the muscle bath was quickly removed, after having checked that neither diastolic tension increased nor spontaneous activity occurred. A container with undercooled liquid propane (–194 °C) – located on the magnetic piston connected to the stimulator – was shut up around the muscle, at a defined moment of the contraction-relaxation cycle. In these experiments the muscles were frozen presystolic, at a moment in which a stimulus would have caused a pronounced contraction.

Diastolic and systolic tension were recorded at high paper velocity during all the operations including impact. In this way any "accident" could be documented by the paper record and the muscle accordingly rejected.

The frozen muscles were then cut with a modified LKB cryoultramicrotome at a temperature of –130 to –140 °C. Ultrathin longitudinal and cross sections were freeze-dried in 10^{-6} torr vacuum and analysed in a Siemens Elmiskop 102 equipped with a Kewex energy dispersive system. (For more details on method see 15).

Electron probe microanalysis

The concentration of an element in the analysed microvolume of a sample is directly related to the ratio between the intensities of specific and unspecific x-ray radiation emitted in the EM from the sample under the electron beam. With the aid of calibration curves – obtained from standards with known elemental composition – absolute concentrations of the elements present in the sample (3), expressed in mmol/kg dry weight, can be calculated. The minimal detectable concentrations with this method are about 2 mmol/kg dry weight for elements such as P, S, Cl, K, Ca. For the low atomic number elements, such as Na, the minimal detectable concentration, due to the lower sensitivity of the detector in this lower energy range is about 20 mmol/kg dry weight. The estimation of low intracellular total calcium concentrations in the presence of high intracellular K concentrations (ca. 500 mmol/kg dry weight) is rendered difficult because of the partial overlap of the $K_{k\beta}$ peak with the $Ca_{k\alpha}$ peak. Accordingly, a deconvolution procedure is adopted in all the reported analyses (for more details see 15).

Results

The heart muscle preparations used in this study developed, under the experimental conditions described above, the full inotropic effect of ouabain within 10 to 30 minutes after application. The smaller strips responded more rapidly. Two strips, each with a diameter of 200 µm, showed the fastest responses.

Diastolic tension did not increase in any of the experiments used for analysis, not even after 1½ hour had elapsed. This indicates that no toxic effects occurred with these doses. The muscle strips being relatively small in diameter, the structural preservation of the most superficial cell layers of muscle enveloped in a thin endocardium was good. The ice crystal damages under these conditions was minimal. It was thus possible to cut at temperatures of −130 to −140 °C ultrathin sections. Therefore small cellular structures such as Z-lines and M-lines in the sarcomeres, mitochondria, t-tubuli, nucleus etc., were identifiable. Altogether, 7 muscle strips were used for analysis.

High sodium concentrations were detected over sarcomeres (Fig. 1a). The concentrations here, were significantly higher than those over the adjacent mitochondria (Fig. 1a). In no other case, neither in muscles frozen in normal diastole, nor in those frozen after other inotropic interventions (Fig. 1b), were similar high sodium concentrations detected.

Potassium concentrations were not as high as in other groups of experiments with muscles frozen in rest (14). However, the concentrations were higher than those in experiments with paired pulse stimulation (Fig. 2b).

The Z-lines and the mitochondria contained little Ca, measured in mmol/kg d.w. This was less than the calcium detected over the sarcomeres (Fig. 1a). The total sarcoplasmic calcium of 6–7 mmol/kg d.w. was higher than that found in other experiments on inotropic interventions (Fig. 2a).

Discussion

Before an attempt can be made to answer the questions asked in the introduction, some comments must be made on the methods used.

1. In studying processes related to relaxation and contraction, physiologists are primarily interested in concentrations of the free ions of a given species, and not in the *total* concentration of an element present in a given cell compartment. With the method used in this study for detecting the elemental concentrations in heart muscle, however, the *total* concentration of an element can be measured – but not the concentration of its free ions. It is important to emphasize this fact in order to avoid any misunderstandings and wrong interpretation of data. Changes in free calcium concentration in cytoplasm during activation and deactivation of contraction *cannot* be detected with electron probe microanalysis: The concentrations of free calcium fluctuates in a range which is under the detectability of the method. On the other hand, in the regulation of relaxation and contraction, storage of calcium in membrane compartments, or/and its release from sites in which it had accumulated, is generally assumed to occur. Moreover, cytoplasmic soluble buffer systems exist and may contribute to the cytoplasmic level of total calcium. Such changes in the total concentration of calcium in specific cell compartments or/and in the sarcoplasm actually can be detected by means of electron probe microanalysis. The

1a

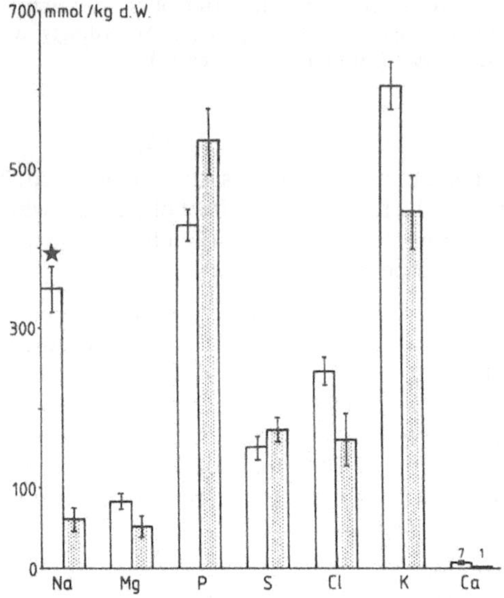

1b

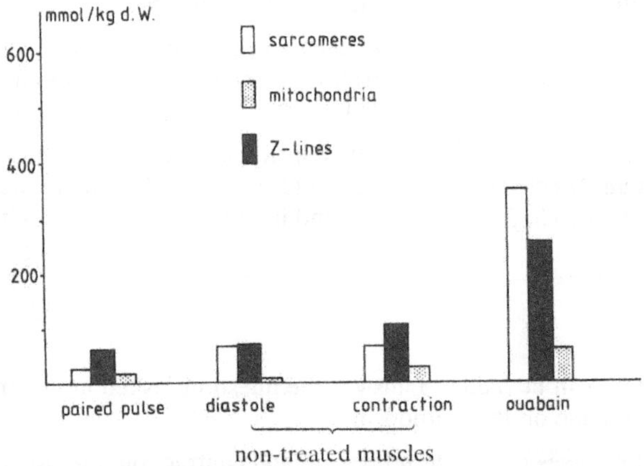

Fig. 1a Presystolic elemental distribution on sarcomeres and adjacent mitochondria in guinea pig heart muscles treated with non-toxic doses of ouabain. The tissue water was removed from the sections by careful freeze-drying at low temperatures and high vacuum. Hence concentrations are given in mmol/kg dry weight. Sarcomeres (No of analysis: 105); mitochondria (No of analyses: 45). Data are means ± S.E. Student's t-test was employed for statistical analysis. Star indicates a $p < 0.01$. Note the significantly higher Na concentration on sarcomeres than in the adjacent mitochondria.

Fig. 1b Intracellular sodium distribution in sarcomeres, mitochondria and Z-lines in muscles frozen in different functional states. The results of the ouabain experiments were summarized, and compared qualitatively with those of published experiments on muscles which had been frozen either after paired pulse stimulation, or during contraction (500 ms after stimulus, at the beginning of the descending flank of the mechanogram), or at the end of diastole in untreated muscle (14, 15).

2a

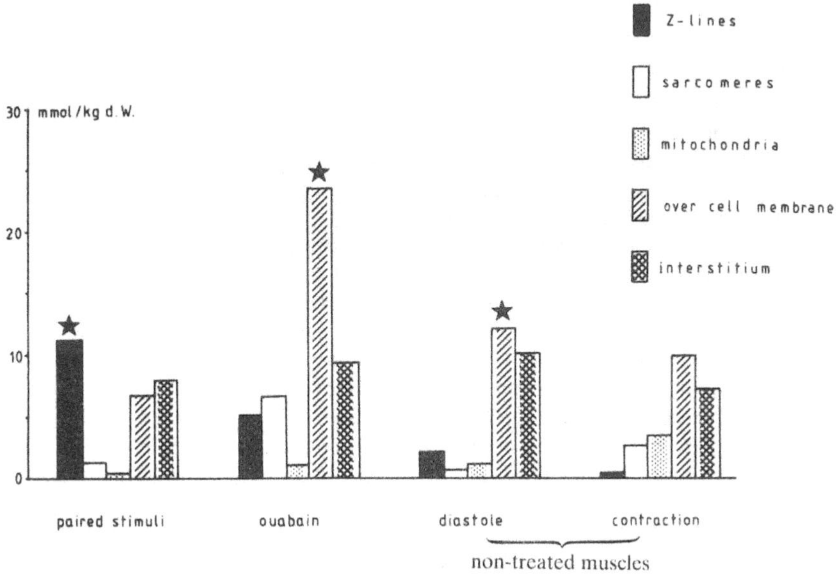

2b

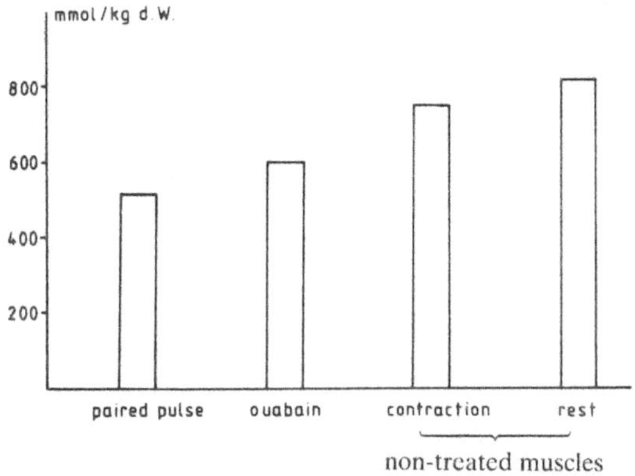

Fig. 2a Calcium distribution in Z-lines, sarcomeres, mitochondria, cell membrane, interstitium in muscles frozen in various functional states. Presystolic Ca-distribution under paired pulse stimulation, ouabain and under control conditions (diastole) as well as during contraction of the non-treated muscle. Stars indicate a significance of $p < 0.01$. T-test was always done between the concentration of Ca in a given compartment (for example mitochondria, cell membrane etc.) and the concentration of Ca in the sarcoplasm. In the ouabain experiments the number of analyses was: 105 on sarcomeres; 45 on mitochondria; 45 over the cell membrane; 20 over the Z-lines. The detailed data of the other summarised experiments have been published (14, 15) or in press elsewhere (15). Under 5mmol/kg dry weight significent differences in Ca concentration are not detectable.

Fig. 2b Potassium concentration in sarcoplasm of muscles frozen after ouabain treatment qualitatively compared with the concentration measured in other published experiments (14, 15).

obtained analytical data give thus information about the cell compartments or cellular buffer systems involved in the accumulation or release of calcium in a particular situation (14).

2. The muscles were prepared for analysis by means of cryotechniques, that is rapid freezing and cryocutting. It is generally assumed that in rapid freezing of biological material, the disadvantage of chemical fixation can be avoided, namely the washing-out of diffusible ions during chemical treatment. It is possible, however, that also during extreme rapid freezing, ionic movements through membranes can take place. This can be the case particularly in the inner region of the tissue, where the rate of freezing inevitably decreases with increasing depth. (These problems have been discussed in detail in other papers (13, 15)). Tests on elemental composition of specific cell compartments in the most superficial layer, and in more internal regions of a muscle, demonstrated the following: At the resolution used for morphology as well as for analysis in the electron microscope, no detectable decrease in the gradients of Ca, and Na concentrations between extra- and intracellular compartments occurred in the outer 10–20 μm of the muscle. The cytoplasmic average concentrations in these superficial cells correspond to that determined otherwise (7, 8, 9).

The most striking finding in these experiments was the high intracellular sodium concentration on the sarcoplasm. This result was characteristic for all the muscles treated with ouabain as well as with k-strophantin (own unpublished experiments). In no other experiments on muscles frozen in other functional states or/and after other positive inotropic interventions were similar high concentrations found over the sarcomeres (Fig. 1b). A lack in the barrier function of the plasma membrane caused by damage which occurred during freezing in deep layers of the tissue could be the cause of diffusion of sodium ions and the accumulation in non normal sites, as well as a loss of intracellular K. But such high concentrations of sodium have never been found even in deeper layer of the tissue, neither in control experiments nor in muscles frozen after other inotropic interventions (Fig. 1b, Fig. 2b). The muscles were treated otherwise identically. Therefore it can be excluded that this finding is an artifact.

This result demonstrates that at non-toxic doses of ouabain a stimulation of the Na^+-K^+ pump can be ruled out under the conditions of our experiments. In the case of stimulation of the pump, an increase in intracellular Na und a decrease in K concentration would not occur.

This finding per se does not demonstrate the *causal* involvement of the Na^+-K^+ pump in the positive inotropic action of ouabain. But it gives evidence that the pump is inhibited at non toxic doses.

In all analysed strips, the highest total calcium accumulation was detected over the cell membrane. It remains to be clarified whether this calcium is bound to structures located externally or internally to the plasmalemma. The concentration of calcium over the interstitium, reflecting the low calcium concentration of the bath solution (1.1 mmol $CaCl_2$), was much lower than that over the cell membrane. If the calcium detected over the cell membrane is bound to structures connected with the external side of the bilayer (glycocalyx-basal lamina) we can expect that lanthanum would displace them. If this calcium is located internally to the bilayer (peripheral components of SR?) it will be also present in preparations in which the glycocalyx-external lamina complex was removed. Future experiments may clarify this point.

The free sarcoplasmic reticulum with its dense rete at the level of the Z-lines in guinea pig heart (14), does not seem to accumulate particularly high concentrations of calcium: the concentrations detected over these regions were not significantly different from that found in normal diastole (Fig. 1a, 2a). Therefore there is no support for the assumption that free SR is especially involved in calcium accumulation under non-toxic doses of ouabain.

High total calcium concentrations were found over the sarcoplasm at the end of diastole. This finding is apparently difficult to reconceil with the complete relaxation of the muscle, which demonstrates that cytoplasmic *free* calcium is low. We detected these high concentrations of *total* calcium in all muscles treated with non-toxic doses of ouabain. This was neither the case in non-treated muscles frozen at the end of normal diastole (Fig. 2a) (15), nor after caffeine treatment (data in preparation), nor after paired pulse stimulation (Fig. 2a) (14). Because of the ability of the muscle to relax completely during diastole, despite the high *total* calcium in the sarcoplasm, it is suggested that a kind of sarcoplasmic buffer system could play some role in maintaining a low cytoplasmic free calcium concentration. This buffer system/s, possibly undergoing conformational changes as a consequence of ouabain treatment, would be able to buffer more Ca^{2+} when its buffer capacity increased with treatment. It remains to be demonstrated whether calmodulin or/and other systems can quantitatively play this role in heart muscle in such situations (1, 12, 16). Electron probe microanalysis would in this case be an interesting "sensor" for the participation of such mechanism in the regulation of sarcoplasmic free Ca^{2+}, by its revealing high levels of *total* intracellular calcium, when relaxation is complete.

The increase in sarcoplasmic calcium as well as sodium can be regarded as a consequence of an inhibition of the Na^+-K^+ pump. As a result of this inhibition, the increase in intracellular Na^+ concentration, involving the Na^+-Ca^{2+} exchange, would lead to the increase in intracellular Ca^{2+}. The amount of this calcium remaining in the ionic form would be an essential factor for the positive inotropic effect of ouabain. This mechanism corresponds essentially to the classical hypothesis of action of cardiac glycosides on heart (5, 10).

The results of these experiments show that, under the described experimental conditions, the participation of this mechanism cannot be excluded and may possibly play a crucial role in the positive inotropic action of cardiac glycosides.

In attempting to answer the questions asked in the introduction, the following conclusions can be made:

1. Intracellular ionic shifts, in this case increase in Na^+ and decrease in K^+ concentrations, have been demonstrated in heart muscle preparations treated with non-toxic doses of ouabain. This finding excludes, at least at these doses, any stimulation of the Na^+-K^+ pump. At the same time, it supports the hypothesis that inhibition of the pump plays an important role in the processes leading to the positive inotropic effects of cardiac glycosides on the myocardium. These results do not rule out other mechanisms which may also play a role in the inotropic action of ouabain at lower doses. An ouabain dependent increase in free catecholamine levels in heart tissue (5) was discussed for the inotropic effect of ouabain at low doses. The participation of this mechanism cannot be excluded until current experiments with reserpinised heart muscles have been completed.
2. Because the existence of sites of calcium accumulation has been demonstrated in these experiments, it is to be expected that experiments in progress will show whether this Ca is mobilised at the very beginning of contraction. That is, at a time at which it can lead to activation of contraction. The described experiments do not give a definite answer to this question.
3. It is possible in heart muscle using x-ray microanalysis to detect structures which clearly accumulate Ca during diastole, after treatment with non-toxic doses of cardiac glycosides. These structures are located near the cell membrane. Moreover, in the sarcoplasm another buffer system is suspected to be involved in Ca binding.

Acknowledgements

The authors would like to thank Mrs. Möller for skillful technical assistance.

Prof. Schlote and Dr. Wolburg from the Department of Submicroscopical Pathology and Neuropathology are kindly acknowledged for their continuous generous support without which this study would have not been possible.

References

1. Fabiato A (1983) Calcium-induced release of calcium from the cardiac sarcoplasmic reticulum. Am J Physiol 245:C1–14
2. Godfraind T, Ghysel-Burton J (1979) Stimulation and inhibition of the sodium pump by cardiotonic steroids in relation to their binding sites and their inotropic effect on guinea-pig isolated atria. Br J Pharmacol 66:175–184
3. Hall TA (1979) Biological x-ray microanalysis. J Microsc 117:145–163
4. Kitazawa T, Shuman H, Somlyo AP (1983) Quantitative electron probe analysis: problems and solutions. Ultramicroscopy 11: 251–262
5. Langer GA (1981) Mechanism of action of the cardiac glycosides on the heart. Biochem Pharmacol 30:3261–3264
6. Noble D (1980) Mechanism of action of therapeutic levels of cardiac glycosides. Cardiovasc Res 14:495–514
7. Page E, Page EG (1968) Distribution of ions and water between tissue compartments in the perfused left ventricle of the rat heart. Circ Res 22:435–46
8. Polimeni PI (1974) Extracellular space and ionic distribution in rat ventricle. Am J Physiol 227:676–683
9. Polimeni PI, Al-Sadir J (1975) Expansion of extracellular space in the non-ischemic zone of the infarcted heart and concomitant changes in tissue electrolyte content in the rat. Circ Res 37:725–732
10. Schwartz A, Lindenmayer GE, Allen JC (1975) The sodium-potassium adenosine triphosphatase: Pharmacological, physiological and biochemical aspects. Pharmacol Rev 27 No 1:3–133
11. Shuman H, Somlyo AV, Somlyo AP (1976) Quantitative electron probe microanalysis of biological thin section: method and validity. Ultramicroscopy 1:317–339
12. Walsh MP, Lepeuch CJ, Vallet B, Cavadore JC, Demaille JG (1980) Cardiac calmodulin and its role in the regulation of metabolism and contraction. J Mol Cell Cardiol 12:1091–1101
13. Wendt-Gallitelli MF, Stöhr P, Wolburg H, Schlote W (1980) Cryoultramicrotomy, electron probe microanalysis and STEM of myocardial tissue. Scanning Electron Microscopy II:499–509
14. Wendt-Gallitelli MF, Jacob R (1982) Rhythm-dependent role of different calcium stores in cardiac muscle: x-ray microanalysis. J Mol Cell Cardiol 14:487–492
15. Wendt-Gallitelli MF, Wolburg H (1984) Rapid freezing, cryosectioning and x-ray microanalysis on cardiac muscle preparation in defined functioned states. J Electron Microscopy Techniques, in press
16. Klee CB, Vanomen TC (1982) Calmodulin. Adv. Protein Chemistry 35:213–321

Authors' address:

Dr. M. F. Wendt-Gallitelli, Physiologisches Institut II, Universität Tübingen, Gmelinstr. 5, 7400 Tübingen

Cardiac glycosides and intracellular Na^+, K^+, Ca^{2+}

E. Noack

Institut für Pharmakologie der Universität Düsseldorf, Düsseldorf (FRG)

Summary

From the fact that cardiac glycosides exert their positiv inotropy most likely via a concentration-dependent inhibition of the Na^+/K^+-activated ATPase, a membrane-bound enzyme regulating the intracellular potassium and sodium homeostasis, one might assume that intracellular electrolyte changes may be easily detectable. Just the opposite holds true. In the literature there are very conflicting observations depending on the experimental model, the analytical method used etc. At the moment, nevertheless, there is great body of evidence that if the cardiac glycoside inotropy is mediated by an inhibition of Na^+/K^+-activated ATPase this is not accompanied by a measurable alteration of intracellar ionic composition. On the other hand toxic concentrations of cardiac glycosides significantly produce a loss of cellular potassium and a rise of cellular sodium and calcium content, especially if arrhythmias are present. The increase of intracellular free and bound calcium, which manifests itself functionally as contracture, is believed to be caused at least by two mechanisms: a stimulation of the Na-Ca-exchange and an inhibition of the specific Ca^{2+}-activated ATPase in the plasma membrane catalyzing the uphill Ca^{2+} outward transport. In vitro studies show that this process is impeded by a local rise of the sodium ion concentration. As the determination of myocardial ion fluxes and cellular electrolyte content has its experimental limitations, further insight may be gained by new techniques which give an answer about possible changes of the electrolyte balance at the subcellular level.

Key words: cardiac glycosides, myocardial electrolyte content, positive inotropic concentrations, toxic electrolyte changes, Ca^{2+} outward transport

It is generally agreed that the Na^+/K^+-activated ATPase is the specific pharmacological receptor for the binding of cardiac glycosides (CG) and for the mediation of their inotropic effects in cardiac muscle. Obviously the main functional role of this membrane-bound enzyme is the maintenance of the intracellular sodium and potassium equilibrium by pumping back sodium ions from the intracellular to the extracellular space and potassium ions vice versa during diastole.

If so, the glycoside-mediated inhibition of this energy-dependent transport process, which is well documented, should result in transient or permanent changes of the cellular electrolyte content of potassium and sodium. As the sodium metabolism on the other hand is intimately linked to the turnover of calcium ions, i.e. by the well-known Na-Ca exchange mechanism, there may be also expected profound influences on intracellular calcium homeostasis as well. In the past, substantial efforts have been undertaken in order to detect possible electrolyte changes in the presence of positive inotropic and toxic concentrations of CG in the myocardial tissue which I would like to summarize briefly in connection with our own experimental efforts to elucidate glycoside-related changes or the cellular ionic composition. As several cellular processes like the aminoacid or sugar transport, which are quite different from the membranous Na^+ and K^+ transport, are nevertheless closely coupled to the activity of the sodium pump, it may be expected that influences of CG on these processes might also indirectly reflect changes of the local interaction at the sarcolemma site.

Looking for possible alterations of the cellular electrolyte content by CG it gives a clearer picture if we separate those effects mediated in the presence of positive inotropic concentrations from those being the consequence of toxic concentrations. An overview of the literature indicates that the findings concerning changes of the cellular K^+ and Na^+ concentration in the isolated heart or atrial preparation exposed to positive inotropic concentrations of CG are inconsistent. Nevertheless, the results of the last years which were performed with a more sophisticated technical equipment are favouring the fact that CG concentrations within the lower therapeutic range do not change significantly the myocardial potassium and sodium content. This is possibly due to the fact that the reserve capacity of the sodium pump coupled to ATPase activity can maintain normal sodium and potassium levels in spite of a moderate inhibition of the pump. On the other hand, there may occur only transient increases in sodium concentration during the contraction period which do not lead to a measurable net accumulation of this ion, as postulated by Akera (1). But in addition there is a great body of evidence that even lower concentrations of CG in a kind of pretherapeutic range may induce a significant increase in cellular K^+ and decrease in cellular Na^+, reflecting a stimulation of the Na^+/K^+ pump. This phenomenon reminds us of the postulate of two different digitalis receptors which may also be involved in this dual effect on myocardial electrolyte content. Up to now a stimulation of the Na-pump by CG, raised for the first time by findings of Carslake and Weatherall (1962), was regarded as an unorthodox hypothesis but it is out of question that an opposite action of low doses of CG to higher doses has been observed in different experimental designs. A representative example are the results of Godfraind and Ghysel-Burton (6) who for 3 hours incubated electrically stimulated guinea-pig left atria in the presence of rising concentrations of ouabain (10^{-9} to 10^{-4} mol/l). Low doses of 10^{-9} and 10^{-8} mol/l ouabain evoked a net increase of intracellular potassium content associated with an equivalent intracellular decrease of sodium concentration, while higher ouabain concentrations in the incubation medium led to a dose – dependent opposite effect. More recently, Bihler and Sawh (2) determined the intracellular Na^+ and K^+ levels of resting and beating guinea-pig left atria. These authors also found a dual effect on the tissue electrolyte content. With a different technique using electrophysiologic measurements, Cohen and co-workers (4) demonstrated an increase of potassium gradient in the presence of low concentrations of ouabain in sheep cardiac Purkinje fibres, and using an ion-sensitive electrode Ellis (5) has observed that concentrations of between 10 and 100 nmol/l ouabain cause a slight decrease in the intracellular sodium activity in Purkinje fibres.

We also extensively studied a possible effect of positive inotropic concentrations of ouabain and digitoxigenin on the cellular potassium and sodium content in isolated electrically driven guinea-pig atria (11, 12). In the presence of clearly positive inotropic concentrations of digitoxigenin (0.6 μmol/l) and two concentrations of ouabain (0.1 and 0.2 μmol/l) we determined a substantial uptake of potassium into the cells and a comparable release of sodium from the tissue in the early phase of inotropy, i.e. in the first three to five minutes after the application of the CG, while the tissue electrolyte content did not differ significantly at the time of maximal positive inotropy. This finding may also reflect a stimulatory effect on the sodium pump which happens transiently if drug concentrations reach a critical level at the receptor site, certainly at an early pretherapeutical concentration level of the CG. Additional experiments lead to the conclusion that the time of maximum effect may be shortened by increasing the frequency of stimulation which may be due to a faster penetration or binding of the CG to the receptor site.

Furthermore, in the presence of a reduced extra-cellular calcium concentration (0.9 mmol Ca^{2+}/l) the ouabain-induced rise in contraction force as well as the time peak of intracellular potassium gain and sodium loss both were markedly delayed although even higher drug concentrations were used in order to get a comparable pharmacological response. The effect must be CG specific, as a positive inotropic concentration of isoproterenol (18 nmol/l) was without any effect on the electrolyte content. This finding also rules out the possibility that an indirect release of catecholamines from their tissue stores might be the reason for the observed electrolyte alterations.

Even in the presence of toxic digitoxigenin concentrations (3.75 μmol/l) the described transient effect of a sodium pump stimulation occurred during the early positive inotropic phase as long as the concentration of CG at the receptor site may be assumed to be relatively low. Also in this case the peak effect occurs more rapidly than in the presence of low CG concentrations. At present it is not clear whether this transient net stimulation of the sodium pump which may be completely dependent on the occasional observation of a stimulation of Na^+, K^+-ATPase in vitro, is in any way linked to the positive inotropic action of CG.

In summary, on the basis of recent studies at least from some experimental efforts it becomes obvious that the positive inotropic action of CG will be preceded by a transient stimulation of the sodium pump, the pharmacological significance of which is still obscure. On the other hand no changes in intracellular potassium and sodium content occur any longer at the time of maximal inotropy.

Concerning the cellular calcium metabolism and turnover it is well established by a lot of experimental results that CG at least in the positive inotropic range increase the amount of exchangeable calcium as well as the intracellular concentration of ionized calcium which often runs in parallel with a significant decrease in total tissue calcium which in our own studies with ouabain piled up to 30% at isolated guinea-pig atria. Several studies using radioactively labelled calcium revealed evidence of an increase in that proportion of the total tissue calcium which could be exchanged with ^{45}Ca. This indicates an increase of calcium exchangeability in the presence of CG which seems to be an unique property of these drugs and which may be partly caused by a profound redistribution of intracellular calcium stores. Only recently, the increase in developed tension occurring concurrently with this increased intracellular availability of ionized calcium was demonstrated by experiments performed by Allen and Blinks (1978). These authors injected aequorin into cells of thin trabeculae from frog atrial muscle and noticed an increase in aequorin-induced light emission following the injection of acetylstrophanthidin.

While in the presence of positive inotropic concentrations of CG many findings as already mentioned are still controversal, the situation is clearer in the presence of toxic concentrations of CG. Numerous studies have shown for human patients as well as for different kinds of animals that toxic concentrations of CG produce a loss of cellular potassium and a rise in cellular sodium content, this certainly as a consequence of an extensive inhibition of Na^+/K^+-ATPase. Obviously the velocity and degree of the electrolyte turnover also depends on the simultaneous occurrence of arrhythmias which accelerate the degree of Na^+ increase in and K^+ loss from the tissue highly significantly.

If toxic concentrations of CG cause a loss of intracellular potassium and an enhanced Na^+ influx it is not difficult to understand why these same concentrations cause a marked increase in Ca^{2+} influx which is completely absent in the presence of therapeutic concentrations. The reason is that Ca^{2+} will enter via two pathways, i.e. in exchange for either intracellular Na^+ or K^+. This leads to an Ca^{2+} overload for the cell and its Ca^{2+} storage sites, yielding an impairment of ATP production, contracture and activation of toxic enzymatic reactions like that of phospholipase activation.

From our own experimental results (Heinen and Noack, 1972) it was interesting to notice that the before mentioned loss of cellular calcium occurring during the initial positive inotropic phase of toxic doses of CG stops just at the moment when inotropy is declining. In contrast it is then turned round to an increase of cellular calcium. At the same time a further exchange of the cellular calcium then is totally prevented. This is certainly due to the fact that

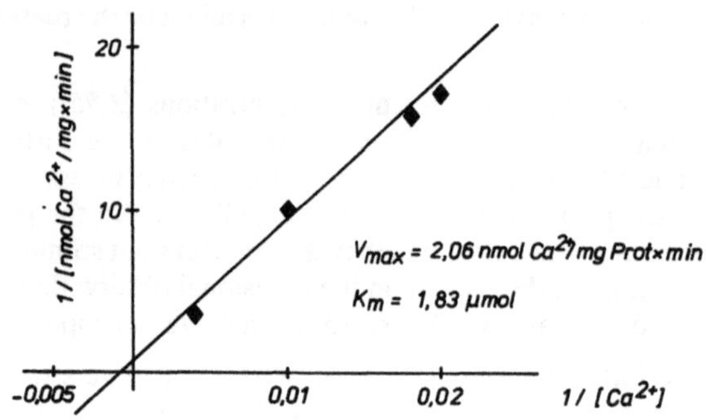

Fig. 1. Kinetics of ATP-dependent Ca^{2+}-uptake into inside-out vesicles of a rabbit sarcolemmal membrane preparation at room temperature.

Ca^{2+} influx into the cell progresses while efflux is completely blocked. From recent work by Caroni and Carafoli (3) there is substantial evidence that calcium ions are actively pumped out by means of an energy-dependent specific Ca^{2+}-ATPase in the myocardium in addition to the well-known Ca-Na-exchange mechanism. The inhibition of this Ca^{2+} transport ATPase by toxic concentrations of CG could then account for the massive calcium overloading seen in the presence of high concentrations. That this process of intoxication is clearly dependent on extracellular calcium may be seen from experiments with isolated, paced Langendorff-perfused rabbit hearts in the presence of a toxic concentration (10 µmol/l) of ouabain. The removal of Ca^{2+} from the extracellular phase allows relaxation to occur in the early stages of the toxic response to the glycosides. But if Ca^{2+} is removed later this intervention remains ineffectual (10).

It is of interest that the specific Ca^{2+} activated ATPase of the plasma membrane which catalyzes the uphill transmembrane Ca^{2+} transport may represent a functional mode of the

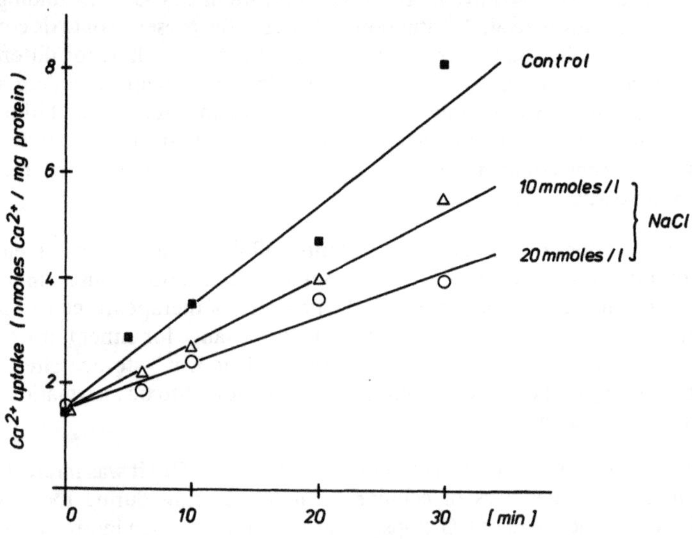

Fig. 2. Inhibition of ATP-dependent Ca^{2+}-uptake at sarcolemmal vesicles by increasing concentrations of sodium chloride in the medium.

Na^+, K^+-ATPase according to a recent publication by Spitzer et al. (13). We, therefore, isolated enzyme-rich vesicles from rabbit ventricular muscle by sucrose gradient centrifugation according to the method of St. Louis and Sulakhe (14) and investigated the influence of increasing ouabain concentrations on the inside-out vesicles which represent the only active configuration. These were separated from the right side out fraction by affinity chromatography, utilizing the carbohydrate-binding characteristics of a wheat germ lectinsepharose column (8).

Figure 1 shows some kinetic characteristics of the calcium pumping enzyme expressed according to the Lineweaver-Burk procedure. Half-maximal activation of the process occurred in the presence of 1.8 µmol/l Ca^{2+}. Maximal transport velocity was relatively low with 2 nmol Ca^{2+}/mg protein × min and tended to decrease further if applying additional purification steps. This ATP-dependent Ca^{2+} uptake was not influenced in the presence of CG. On the contrary, rising concentrations of sodium caused an increasing inhibition as shown in figure 2. Therefore, we think it possible that the elevation of the local sodium concentration near the plasmalemma site as a consequence of CG-induced inhibition of the Na^+/K^+-ATPase may account for the observed inhibition of Ca^{2+}-efflux after the application of toxic glycoside concentrations. This is perhaps also an explanation for the finding by Nayler and Williams (9) that Ca^{2+} overloading caused by the administration of toxic doses of CG precedes the decline of the tissure stores of ATP in marked contrast to the biochemical alterations which occur in hypoxic heart muscle.

In conclusion it is out of discussion that toxic concentrations of CG cause marked and easily detectable changes in the electrolyte content of heart muscle which are a logical result of a pronounced inhibition of the Na^+/K^+-activated ATPase and coupled Na^+ pump, respectively. The observed alterations involve a gain in Na^+ and Ca^{2+} and a loss of K^+. In contrast, it seems unlikely that this same mechanism provides the basis for the positive inotropic effect of the CG, unless we assume that the degree of inhibition is so moderate that it does not bring about measurable electrolyte changes. This could go in parallel with an altered cellular distribution and exchangeability of the physiological important electrolytes resulting in a regional accumulation that favours E-C-coupling. Last not least, it must be admitted that the determination of the total tissue electrolyte content has its disadvantages giving very limited information about the local cellular situation and electrolyte homeostasis because that portion of free ionic concentration which is of biological significance remains unknown. In addition any cellular electrolyte compartmentation for example at the plasmalemmal site remains obscure.

References

1. Akera T, Bennett RT, Olgaard MK, Brody MK (1976) Cardiac Na^+, K^+-adenosine triphosphatase inhibition by ouabain and myocardial sodium: a computer simulation. J Pharmacol Exp Ther 199:287–297
2. Bihler I, Sawh PC (1979) Regulation of sugar transport in the myocardium. Effects of ouabain in resting and beating isolated guinea-pig left atria. J Mol Cell Cardiol 11:407–414
3. Caroni P, Carafoli E (1980) An ATP-dependent Ca^{2+}-pumping system in dog heart sarcolemma. Nature 283:765–767
4. Cohen I, Daut J, Noble D (1976) An analysis of the actions of low concentrations of ouabain on membrane currents in Purkinje fibres. J Physiol (London) 260:75–103
5. Ellis D (1977) The effect of external cations and ouabain on the intracellular sodium activity of sheep heart Purkinje fibres. J Physiol (London) 273:211–240
6. Godfraind T, Ghysel-Burton J (1977) Binding sites related to ouabain-induced stimulation or inhibition of the sodium pump. Nature (London) 265:165–166
7. Heinen E, Noack E (1972) Effects of k-strophanthin and digitoxigenin on contractile force, calcium content and exchange in guinea-pig isolated atria. Naunyn-Schmiedeberg's Arch Exp Path Pharm 275:359–371

8. Mas-Oliva J, Williams A, Nayler WG (1980) Two orientations of isolated cardiac sarcolemmal vesicles separated by affinity chromatography. Anal Biochem 103:222–226
9. Nayler W, Williams A (1978) Relaxation in heart muscle: some morphological and biochemical considerations. Eur J Cardiol 7:Suppl. 35–50
10. Nayler W, Noack E (1981) Influence of cardiac glycosides on electrolyte exchange and content in cardiac muscle cells. In: "Handbook of Experimental Pharmacology" Vo. 56/I, "Cardiac Glycosides". Greeff K Ed p 407–436 (Springer Verlag, Berlin)
11. Noack E, Felgenträger J, Zettner B (1979) Changes in myocardial Na and K content during development of cardiac glycoside inotropy. J Mol Cell Cardiol 11:1189–1194
12. Noack E, Felgenträger J, Zettner B (1978) Kinetics of changes in K^+-, Na^+- and Ca^{2+}-content in heart tissue in the presence of cardiac glycosides. Naunyn Schmiedeberg's Arch Pharmacol 302:R 34
13. Spitzer E, Grosse R, Kuprijanov V, Preobrazhensky A (1981) Demonstration of a digitalis-sensitive sarcolemmal Ca^{2+}-pump functionally coupled with a membrane associated creatine phosphokinase. Acta biol med germ 40:1111–1122
14. St. Louis PJ, Sulakhe PV (1976) Adenosine triphosphate-dependent calcium binding and accumulation by guinea-pig cardiac sarcolemma. Can J Biochem 54:946–956

Author's address:

Prof. Dr. E. Noack, Institut f. Pharmakologie d. Universität Düsseldorf, Universitätsstraße 1, 4000 Düsseldorf

Cardiac glycosides with different effects in the heart

H. Lüllmann, T. Peters, H.-H. Prillwitz, and A. Ziegler

Department of Pharmacology, University of Kiel, Kiel (FRG)

Summary

Remarkable differences exist between the effects of different cardiac glycosides (native and semisynthetic) with respect to the affinity and to the magnitude of inotropic responses and their time courses. At glycoside concentrations which lead to identical Na-K-ATPase inhibitions, the inotropic responses vary widely. This finding contradicts the hypothesis that the increase of contractile force is the consequence of an ATPase inhibition and causally related to it.

We propose the hypothesis that the inhibition of ATPase and the inotropic stimulation provoked by cardiac glycosides are two parallel events, not causally related but both mediated by the same receptor. The inhibition of the Na-K-ATPase is the consequence of the occupation and thus proportional to the concentration of the glycoside-ATPase complexes. In contrast, the inotropic response is determined by the frequency of glycoside-ATPase-interactions. Glycosides which possess high association and dissociation rate constants will interact with the ATPase with high frequencies and thus will evoke larger inotropic responses at a given ATPase inhibition than glycosides with low turnover rates.

Key words: cardiac glycosides – ATPase inhibition – inotropic response – occupation – turnover rate

Introduction

The effect of cardiac glycosides on isolated heart muscle preparations can be described by four parameters: the affinity, the maximal extent by which the contractile force can increase, the rate of onset of the inotropic response and the rate by which the response declines upon wash-out of the drug, and finally the occurrence of toxic signs (arrhythmia and increase of resting tension). When studying different glycosides under identical standardized conditions, great differences can be observed between the various compounds with respect to the above parameters. This is demonstrated for some glycosides in Fig. 1. The concentrations are chosen to obtain a maximum of inotropism without signs of intoxication after time periods long enough to warrant an effect equilibrium.

The slow development of the action of the conventional glycosides and the poor reversibility allows the testing of only one dose per isolated organ. Dose response curves based on one dose per organ are shown in Fig. 2. This set of curves clearly demonstrates that the investigated glycosides differ over a wide range not only with respect to their affinities but also with respect to the maximum extent of inotropism. Applying pharmacological terms, one could speak of different intrinsic activities of the cardiac glycosides.

Proscillaridin A for example enhanced the contractile force by about 20% only; this concentration (3×10^{-8}M) already induced arrhythmia in 6 out of 10 experiments. In contrast, 3-β-OH-4,5-methylene-AB-trans-scillarenin, also possessing a high affinity, increased the contractile force by more than 100% without any signs of toxicity. The "classical" glycoside ouabain induced an inotropic effect of about 65%, the next higher concentration was no longer tolerated. The semisynthetic glycoside 3-α-methyl-digitoxigenin glucoside with low affinity increased the contractile force again by 80–100%. From this quantitative evaluation we can conclude that striking differences exist between the individual glycosides with respect

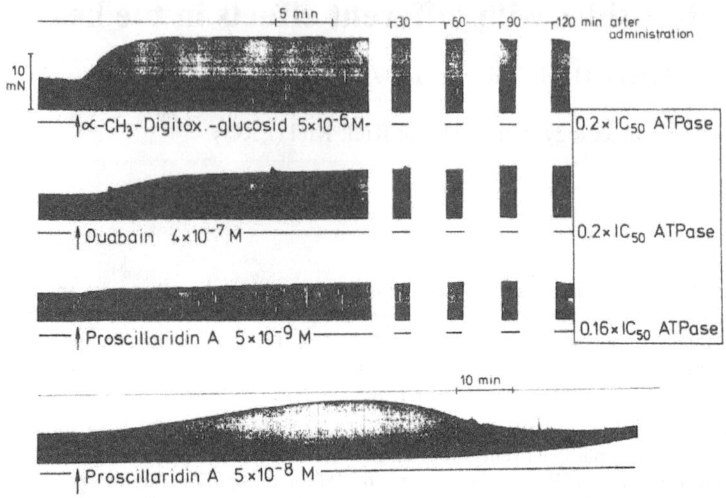

Fig. 1. Mechanograms of isolated electrically driven (3 Hz) guinea-pig atria. Three glycosides were applied in concentrations corresponding to 0.2 times the half maximal inhibition of Na-K-ATPase (IC_{50}). Note the differences in the time courses of the effects and their magnitudes (upper three curves). The comparably small inotropic effect of proscillaridin A can be enhanced by a higher concentration but this response is transient and followed by intoxication.

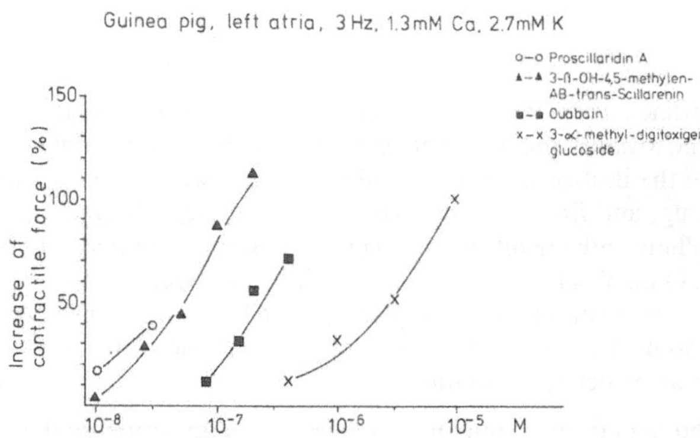

Fig. 2. Dose response curves of two native and of two semisynthetic cardiac glycosides. Each point is the mean of 6–10 experiments. Only one dose was applied per isolated left atrium, the effect was observed for 2 hours. The dose response curves are limited since at higher concentrations toxic signs occurred.

to the inotropic maximum which can be attained without development of toxic signs even after long periods of exposure. These differences, which can be demonstrated by a method as simple as recording the mechanograms, prompted us to search for an explanation of the different inotropic activities of cardiac glycosides.

To obtain information on the electrolyte content of atrial tissue exposed to different concentrations of different glycosides, the potassium and sodium contents were determined after 75 min of incubation. The results of two experiments are depicted in Fig. 3 in relation to the mechanical dose response curves. In case of proscillaridin A, the concentration 10^{-8}M induced about 15 % increase of contractile force and left the K- and Na-contents unaltered. But already the concentration 3×10^{-8}M induced a marked loss of K and a gain of Na, accompanied by an inotropic response of about 30 % and toxic signs in half of the preparations. The higher concentration 10^{-7}M provoked only a transient increase of contractile force and led to intoxication in all cases; the changes of the cellular electrolyte concentrations were still more pronounced. The threshold concentration of 3-β-OH-4,5-methylen-AB trans-scillarenin is almost comparable with that of proscillaridin A. 3×10^{-8}M enhanced the contractile force by about 30 %. At a concentration of 10^{-7}M the contractile force was increased by about 85 %, the K- and Na-contents of tissue were found unchanged. Even the next higher concentration, 3×10^{-7}M 3-β-OH-4,5-methylen-AB trans-scillarenin, was tolerated and brought the contractile force up to about 110 % being accompanied though by a loss of K and a gain of Na. From these results and from the outcome of additional experiments with other native and semisynthetic glycosides, we can conclude that there is no correlation between the extent of inotropism and the impairment of the cellular K- and Na-concentrations; on the other hand there is a close correlation between the electrolyte impairment and toxicity. The first changes of the cellular electrolyte composition occur at very different degrees of inotropism.

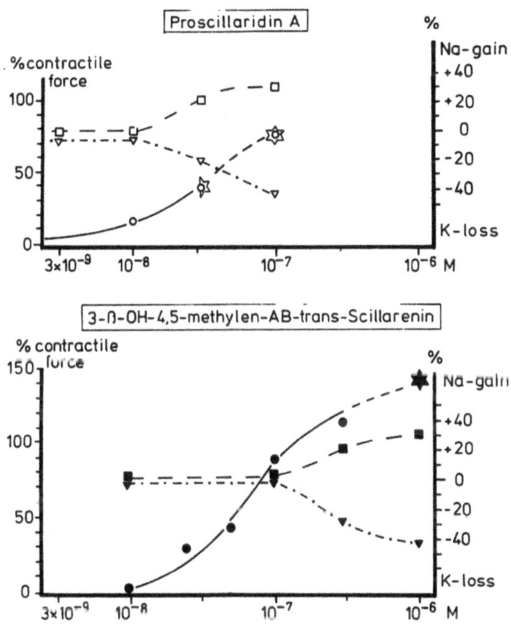

Fig. 3. Influence of proscillaridin A and of 3-β-OH-4,5-methylene-AB-trans-scillarenin upon the Na and K contents of isolated, beating guinea-pig atria. The muscles were exposed for 75 minutes to the glycosides at different concentrations (abscissa). The alterations of the electrolyte concentrations are indicated as percentage changes on the right ordinate. The increases of contractile forces (solid lines) are indicated in percentage on the left ordinate. The glycoside concentrations which evoked toxic signs are marked by asterisk symbols. Note: In case of proscillaridin A an impairment of the ion gradients at the concentration of 3×10^{-8}M is accompanied by an increase of the contractile force of about 30 % (6 out of 10 atria already displayed intoxication) whereas a comparable ionic impairment induced by the semisynthetic glycoside (3×10^{-7}M) is accompanied by an inotropic response of more than 100 % (C. Beyer, 1984; H. Wulf, 1984).

Since the impairment of the K and Na gradients is thought to be the consequence of an inhibition of the Na-K-ATPase, we studied the K-pump function of atrial tissue at different concentrations of the respective glycosides. The results obtained with four different glycosides are summarized in Fig. 4. In the upper part the mechanical dose response curves are shown, the lower part demonstrates the dose-dependent inhibition of the K transport. Equieffective concentrations of the glycosides, which reduce the K transport by 20% (dashed horizontal line), are projected onto the mechanical dose response curves. As can be seen from the graph, the 20% K-transport inhibition coincides with greatly differing degrees of inotropism: for proscillaridin A 20% transport inhibition corresponds to about 20%, for ouabain to about 30%, and for the two semisynthetic glycosides to 70–80% increase of contractile force. This result suggests that the magnitude of the inotropic response is not correlated with the degree of ATPase inhibition.

So far the reported results do not provide an explanation of the differences between the individual glycosides. Nevertheless they demonstrate that there is not a simple correlation between Na-K-ATPase occupation and the inotropic response. To come back to the mechanograms (Fig. 1), another parameter which has not been considered so far seems to call for attention, i.e., the rates of onset of the inotropic effect. It seems remarkable that those

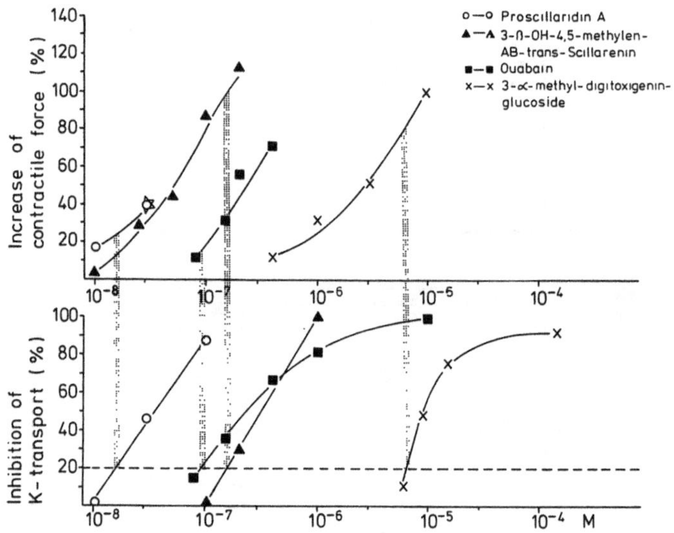

Fig. 4. Influence of two native and of two semisynthetic glycosides upon the K-transport capability of isolated, beating guinea-pig atria. In the upper part, dose-response-curves of the increase of contractile force are depicted (compare Fig. 2). In the lower part the inhibition of the K-transport is demonstrated as percentage of controls. The 20% level of inhibition is indicated by the horizontal dashed line. For each glycoside the 20% inhibition is projected upward on the dose-response-curve of inotropism (stippled lines). Note: In case of proscillaridin A and of ouabain the 20% inhibition of K transports coincides with small increases of contractile force, while the same transport inhibition occurs only at inotropic levels of 80–100% in case of the semisynthetic glycosides.
The K transport was estimated in the following way: after 75 minutes of exposure to the glycosides in a Tyrode solution containing 2.7 mM K, the K concentration was raised for 15 minutes to 7.4 mM and the K content of the tissue determined by flame photometry. The transport capability of glycoside treated heart muscles were compared with that of untreated controls which took up 8–10 mmoles K per kg wet weight. (C. Beyer, 1984; H. Wulf, 1984).

glycosides (e.g. proscillaridin A) which display a narrow mechanical dose-response-curve and an overproportional degree of ATPase inhibition show a very slow rate of onset, whereas the semisynthetic glycosides which are characterized by a broad dose-response-curve, by a great magnitude of inotropic response, and by an underproportional ATPase inhibition possess a fast rate of onset and of offset of the inotropic response. The different rates cannot be explained by disposition kinetics; they rather point to differences at the receptor level. We therefore studied the binding kinetics of different glycosides by using a cardiac Na-K-ATPase preparation and applying two complementary methods: 1.) Continuous determination of ATP hydrolysis, addition of a certain glycoside concentration, determination of the time course to reach the decreased hydrolysis rate; 2.) Observation of the time course of binding of radiolabelled glycosides to the ATPase, and of the time course of release due to competition by high concentrations of unlabelled glycoside. This approach allowed us to evaluate the association rate constant (k_{+1}), the dissociation rate constant (k_{-1}), and the dissociation constant ($K_D = \frac{k_{-1}}{k_{+1}}$). It is obvious that those glycosides which induce slow mechanical response display low association rates and dissociation rates and vice versa. This is shown also by means of radioactive labelled glycosides (Fig. 5): 3-α-methyl-digitoxigenin-glucoside reached its binding equilibrium much faster than ouabain and was released more rapidly than ouabain.

What is the significance at the receptor level of such very different rate constants?
1. Obviously, the dissociation constants are stationary values and do not provide information concerning the turnover rate of the drug-receptor-complex formation. To illustrate this, a set of ATPase-inhibition curves is depicted in Fig. 6 and relative turnover rates are indicated. At any given level of inhibition the relative turnover rates vary between 0.5 and <44. Thus, in

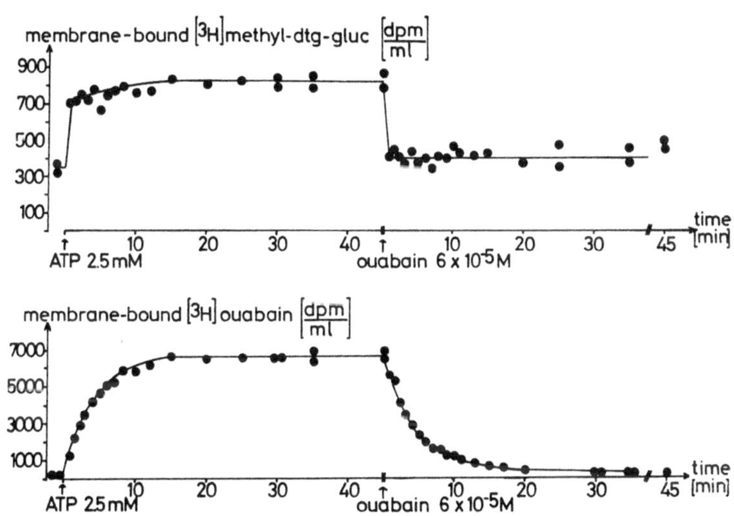

Fig. 5. Binding and release of 3-α-methyl-digitoxigenin-glucoside and of ouabain by and from a Na-K-ATPase preparation of guinea-pig ventricular muscle. The concentrations of the two compounds were chosen to obtain a half maximal occupation of the Na-K-ATPase. The reaction was started by addition of ATP, the release was induced by addition of unlabelled ouabain (6×10^{-5}M). Note the different time courses. A quantitative analysis of the result yielded the following values: Ouabain $k_{+1} = 1.9 \times 10^4$, $k_{-1} = 3.4 \times 10^{-3}$, the semisynthetic glycoside $k_{+1} = 4.6 \times 10^4$, M^{-1} sec^{-1} and $k_{-1} = 100 \times 10^{-3}$ sec, respectively. For details see Mohr, 1983.

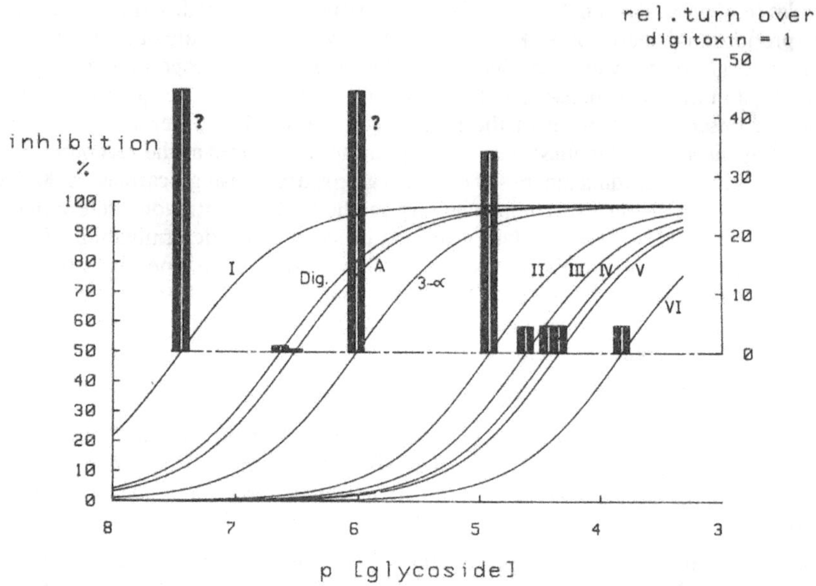

Fig. 6. Concentration dependent inhibition by different glycosides of cardiac Na-K-ATPase. The individual curves are calculated on the basis of experimentally determined IC_{50} values. The attached bars indicate turnover rates, the turnover rate of digitoxin = 1. The turnover rates are calculated from the associations and dissociations occurring per unit of time: $k_{+1} \times [G] \times [ATPase_2] = k_{-1} \times [G\text{-}ATPase_2]$ under equilibrium conditions.
The inhibition curves consist of stationary values which do not provide information on the frequencies of interactions. The turnover rates vary in a wide range and are independent of the concentrations which led to half maximum inhibition; compare the relative turnover rates of digitoxin and acetylgitoxin (A) with those of compound I and 3-α-Scillarenin (3-α).
I 3-β-Hydroxy-4,5-methylene-AB-trans-scillarenin
II 3-α-Ethinyl-digitoxigenin mono-rhamnoside
III 3-α-Methyl-digitoxigenin mono-glucoside
IV 3-α-Methyl-digitoxigenin mono-rhamnoside
V 3-α-Methyl-β-hydroxy-digitoxigenin
VI 3-β-Methyl-α-hydroxy-digitoxigenin

case of a "slow glycoside" only very few associations and dissociations occur per unit of time; for a "fast glycoside" the frequency of association and dissociation may be hundred fold higher, while inducing an identical degree of ATPase inhibition.

2. It is also obvious that the dissociation rate constant determines the mean life time of the glycoside ATPase complex. In case of the classical glycosides the life time of the complex is rather long, i.e., in the order of minutes. It depends on the experimental conditions and is species dependent.

3. Furthermore the rate constants determine the time course of attaining the equilibrium binding. This is demonstrated for an ATPase preparation in which the disposition does not play a role and for an isolated heart muscle preparation in which the disposition of the drug retards the time course (Fig. 7).

From the foregoing reported results we are left with the following problems. Under the assumption that both biological effects of cardiac glycosides are induced by specific binding to one receptor site, i.e., the Na-K-ATPase, two different relations can be deduced:

1. For any given level of ATPase inhibition, the occupation of ATPase molecules is identical for all glycosides, whereas the turnover rates (the frequencies of interactions) vary over a wide range.
2. For any given magnitude of inotropism, the frequency of glycoside-ATPase-interaction seems to be identical, whereas the occupation varies widely.

The consequence of these two relations is that the inotropic response can be dissociated from the degree of ATPase inhibition. It appears, therefore, unreasonable to causally relate the glycoside-induced increase of contractile force with an inhibition of the Na-K-ATPase.

We think the mode of action of cardiac glycosides should be re-considered. The two effects, inhibition and inotropism, are parallel events rather than being consecutive events causally related to each other. The degree of ATPase inhibition is simply determined by the

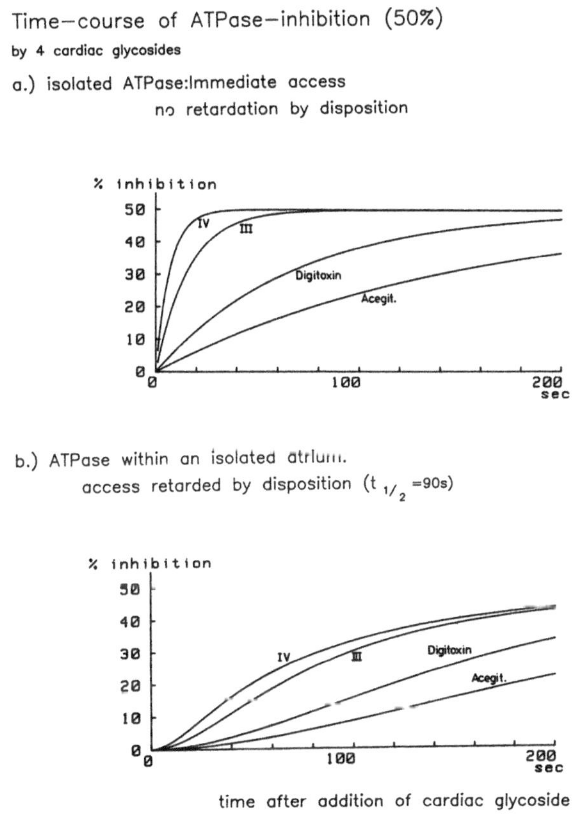

Fig. 7. Time courses of inhibition of the Na-K-ATPase by glycosides with different rate constants. The concentrations of the four glycosides are chosen to obtain half maximum inhibition. In the upper part the time courses of inhibition are depicted for an isolated ATPase preparation in which the inhibitor has immediate access to its binding sites. In the lower part the same process is simulated for an isolated organ. In this case the disposition within the extracellular space retards the onset of inhibition. Abbreviations s. Fig. 6.

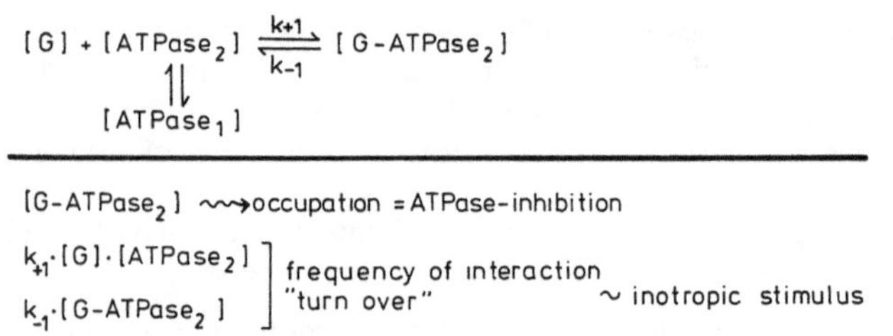

Fig. 8. Kinetic model describing the interaction of a cardiac glycoside (G) with a certain conformation of the Na-K-ATPase which occurs during a pump cycle ($ATPase_2$), k_{+1} and k_{-1} association and dissociation rate constants, respectively. The interactions are thought to lead to two consequences: 1.) the concentration of the glycoside-ATPase-complexes ($G\text{-}ATPase_2$) or occupation determines the inhibition of the ATPase; 2.) each interaction provides an inotropic stimulus, the frequency of interactions determines the inotropic response. During equilibrium $k_{+1} \times [G] \times [ATPase_2]$ equals $k_{-1} \times [G\text{-}ATPase_2]$.

occupation of ATPase molecules per unit of time: it is the sum of occupied ATPase molecules, independent of whether a small fraction is complexed for a long time or a large fraction for a short time. In contrast, the inotropism is dependent on the frequency at which cardiac glycosides interact with the ATPase receptor. A cardiac glycoside molecule produces an inotropic stimulus when interacting with its binding site thereby preserving a particular conformation of the Na-K-ATPase. The cardiac glycosides can, therefore, be considered as

1. inhibitors of the Na-K-ATPase, and
2. agonists mediating inotropic stimuli.

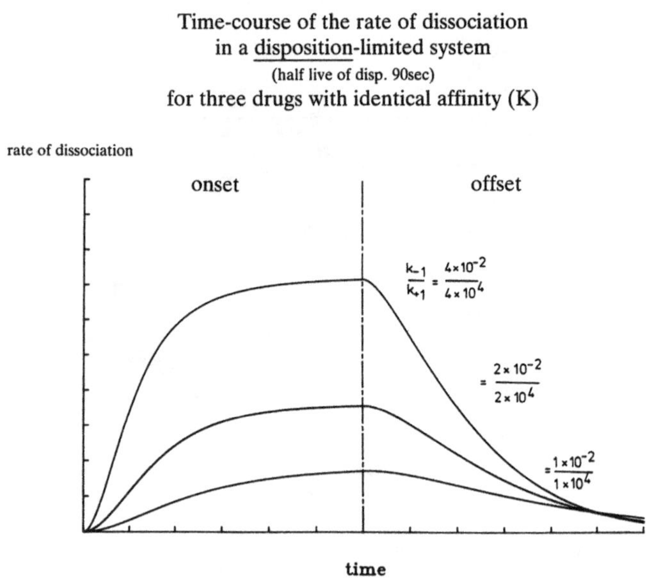

Fig. 9. Theoretical curves demonstrating the frequency of dissociation ($k_{-1} \times [G\text{-}ATPase_2]$) after addition and after wash-out (vertical line) of three glycosides with different rate constants but identical affinities (K_D). The disposition is taken into account with a half life time of 90 sec. The three glycosides induce identical levels of ATPase inhibition, but different time courses and magnitudes of "inotropic responses" if the rate of dissociation is considered to be the inotropic stimulus.

This concept can formally be described as shown in Fig. 8. To illustrate the significance which the turnover rates have for the magnitude of the inotropic response, the corresponding curves have been calculated using the kinetic data obtained by the experiments described above. In Fig. 9 the time courses and the magnitudes of the inotropic responses of different glycosides are depicted. At concentrations which lead to identical occupation of the Na-K-ATPase, the time courses and the magnitudes of "inotropic responses" vary greatly. These calculated inotropic responses are similar to those from the recorded mechanograms.

We conclude that the positive inotropic effect of cardiac glycosides is determined by the frequency of interaction with the Na-K-ATPase. This hypothesis allows the description of the pharmacological events and their time courses, and it readily explains the dissociation between the inotropic response and the impairment of Na- and K-gradients. It remains, however, an open question, which molecular event is responsible for the stimulus. Is it the formation of the glycoside-ATPase complex or the dissociation of the complex, or both?

References

1. Beyer C (1984) Der Einfluß toxischer Konzentrationen von g-Strophanthin und 3-α-Methyldigitoxigenin-β-glucosid auf den Natrium- und Kaliumhaushalt der Herzmuskelzelle. Dissertation, Med Fakultät, Kiel
2. Mohr K (1983) Kinetics of binding of the semi-synthetic α-methyl-digitoxigenin-glucoside to cardiac Na^+-K^+-ATPase. Biochem Pharmacol 32:928–930
3. Wulf H (1984) Zum Einfluß halbsynthetischer Digitoxigenin- und Scillarenin-Derivate auf Kontraktions-Kraft, Natrium-Kalium-Gehalt und Kaliumtransport isolierter linker Meerschweinchen-Vorhöfe. Dissertation, Med Fakultät, Kiel

Authors' address:

Dr. Heinz Lüllmann, Abt. f. Pharmakologie Universität Kiel, Hospitalstr. 4–6, 2300 Kiel

Biphasic positive inotropic actions of ouabain on rat, guinea-pig and cat heart: a mathematical description

J. M. Koomen, W. H. van Gilst, J. A. M. Schevers, and J. Wilting

Faculty of Pharmacy, Department of Pharmacology, State University of Utrecht, Utrecht (The Netherlands)

Summary

The inotropic action of ouabain on isolated perfused hearts of rat, guinea-pig, and cat was studied over a wide concentration range (10^{-12}-5×10^{-3} M). In all three species used, the positive inotropic effect (PIE) of ouabain appeared to be biphasic in character. However, there was a remarkable difference in the course of the logdose-response curves of ouabain on guinea-pig and cat heart as compared with than on rat heart. The first two species showed, at very low concentrations of ouabain (guinea-pig heart: 10^{-9} M and cat heart: 10^{-10} M), a typical bell-shaped increase in cardiac contractile activity, while at higher concentrations (10^{-8}-10^{-6} M and 10^{-9}-10^{-7} M, respectively) the normally observed S-shaped increase in contractile activity occurred. On the contrary, rat hearts showed a flat S-curve between 10^{-8} and 10^{-6} M and a steep one between 10^{-6} and 10^{-4} M of ouabain. In order to explain the biphasic action of ouabain a hypothetical model for the mechanism(s) of action of ouabain is discussed. Mathematical description of this model is based on the existence of two different receptor-types for ouabain. It is suggested that sarcolemmal-bound calcium may play an important role in both mechanisms of inotropic action of ouabain.

Key words: ouabain, inotropy, heart, rat, guinea-pig, cat

Introduction

Since von Loewie in 1917 described a remarkable similarity between the positive inotropic action of ouabain and calcium ions, many theories have been postulated to explain the mechanism of action of cardiac glycosides. Although an inhibition of the sarcolemmal Na^+/K^+-pump as a cause of positive inotropic activity of the heart is very likely (Akera and Brody, 1977), many investigators seem to be convinced of the existence of a second type of action which, on the contrary, is linked with a stimulation of the monovalent cation pump (Askari, 1971; Lee and Klaus, 1971; Peters et al., 1974; Blood, 1975; Cohen et al., 1976; Godfraind and Ghysel-Burton, 1977; Okita, 1977). Important evidence for the existence of two different mechanisms of actions comes from studies which demonstrate the presence of two receptor-types for cardiac glycosides (Lüllmann and Ravens, 1973; Gervais et al., 1977; Heller and Beck, 1978; Ghysel-Burton and Godfraind, 1979; De Pover and Godfraind, 1979). In the study presented here, we administered ouabain to isolated stimulated hearts of rat, guinea-pig and cat over a wide concentration range (10^{-12} M-5×10^{-3} M).

Methods

Male Wistar rats (200–300 g) and male random bred guinea-pigs and cats were anesthetized with diethylether. After heparinization the thorax was opened, the aorta cannulated and the heart quickly removed. Subsequently the heart was perfused according to Langendorff at a constant perfusion pressure (8 kPa) and temperature (37 °C). The standard salt solution ($CaCl_2$ = 1.36 mM) was saturated with a 95 % O_2–5 % CO_2-gas mixture (pH = 7.35 ± 0.05). After removal of the atria and dissection of the mitral valve,

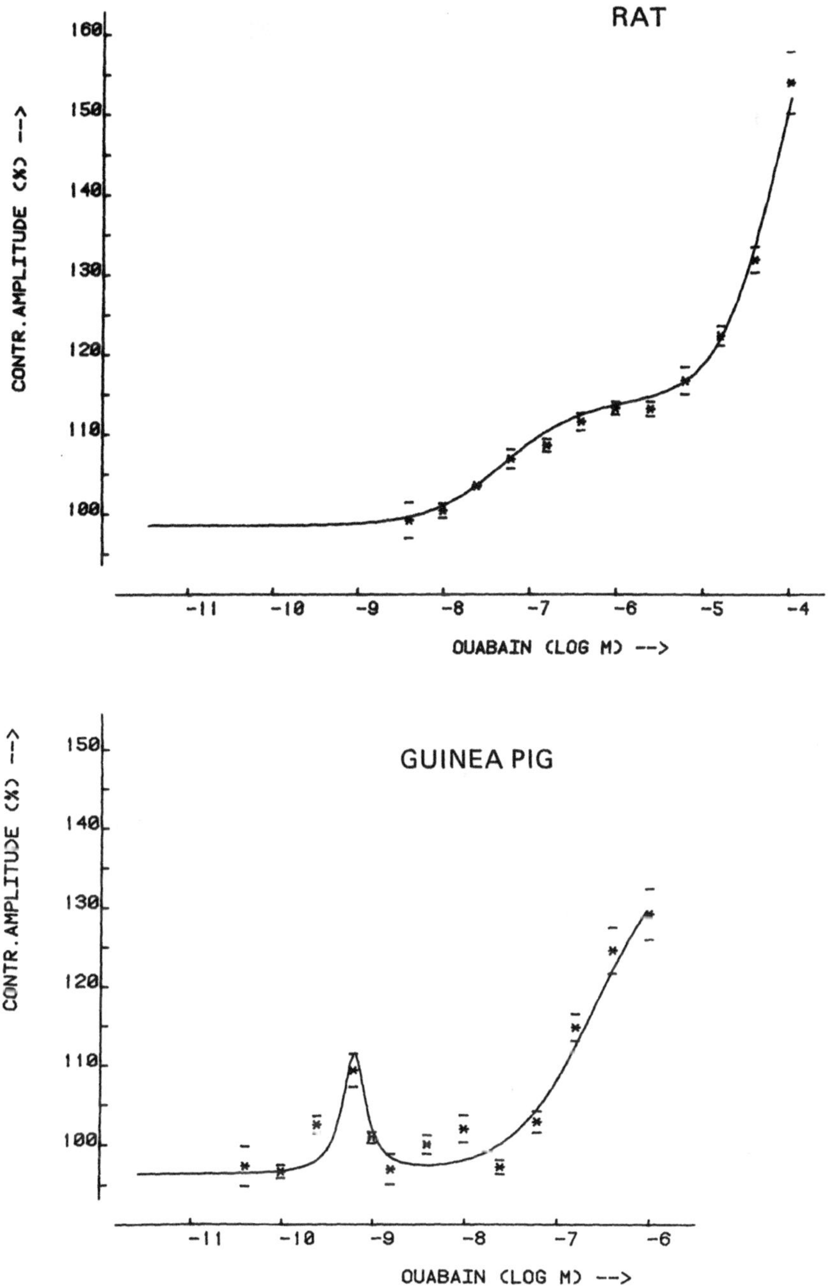

Fig. 1. Experimental data (mean ± s.e.m.) of ouabain-induced positive inotropy and theoretical logdose-response curves (solid lines are computer read-outs, see Discussion) of ouabain on isolated heart of rat (Ia; r = 0.9956), guinea-pig (Ib; r = 0.9165) and cat (Ic).

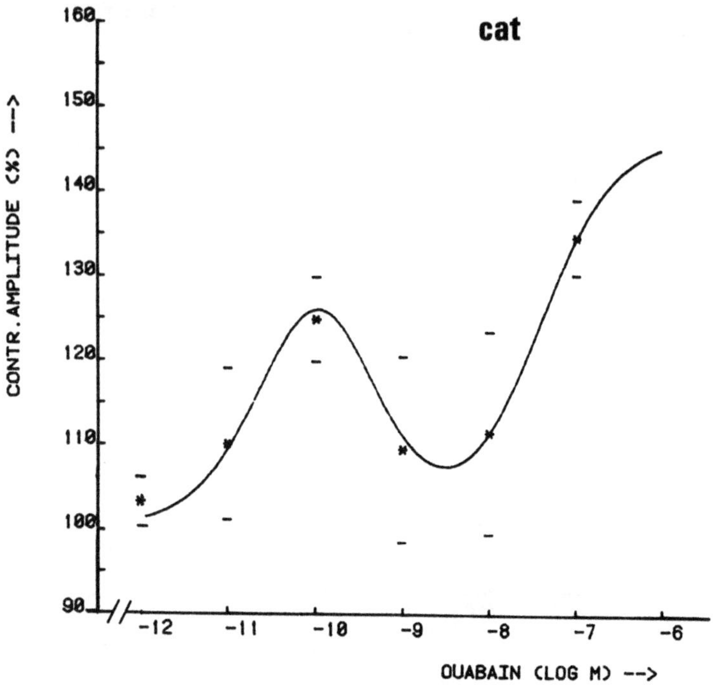

the heart was stimulated electrically (300 beats per minute; 6 V/3 ms). Contraction amplitude was measured by recording apico-basal shortening of the heart isotonically with a displacement transducer. Changes in contraction amplitude were expressed as percentages of the preceding control values (= 100%). Coronary flow was measured manually throughout the experiment. Perfusion sequence was as follows: after a stabilization period of 40 minutes, the heart was perfused during 6 min with a ouabain-solution in order to obtain a stable inotropic effect. Each heart was treated successively with five different concentrations of ouabain which were applied in random order. Intermediate wash-out periods (standard salt solution) of 8 minutes were sufficient to restore normal control values for contractility. Differences between means were regarded as significant when p-values were ≤ 0.05 (two-sided Student t-test).

Results

Isolated rat heart: The biphasic PIE of ouabain on rat heart is shown in figure Ia. Between 10^{-8} and 10^{-6} M ouabain contraction amplitude increased significantly. The "first" PIE reached a maximum value of about 15% above control at 10^{-6} M ouabain. A "second", clearly distinguishable, PIE of ouabain occurred between 10^{-6} and 10^{-4} M ouabain. This second part of the logdose-response curve was in full agreement with data from literature (see Discussion). Concentrations of ouabain higher than 10^{-4} M induced arrythmia, contracture and heart block.

Isolated guinea-pig heart: Ouabain concentrations between 10^{-10} and 10^{-8} M gave a typical bell-shaped increase in cardiac contractile activity (see figure Ib). This increment appeared to be significant (2.5×10^{-10} M: $p \leq 0.05$ and 6.25×10^{-10} M: $p \leq 0.001$) and the maximum PIE was 10% above control. At higher concentrations (10^{-9} to 2.5×10^{-8} M ouabain) this "first" PIE disappeared. However, between 10^{-8} and 10^{-6} M ouabain the well-known sigmoid-shaped logdose-response curve of ouabain on contractile activity was obtained. Concentrations of ouabain above 10^{-6} M induced arrhythmia, contracture and heart block.

Isolated cat heart: The PIE of ouabain on cat heart contractility (see figure Ic) was comparable with the results described for guinea-pig heart. Cat hearts, however, appeared to be more sensitive to ouabain and responded in a more pronounced increment in contractile activity at the lowest concentrations tested (10^{-11}–10^{-10} M). The limited number of cat hearts available forced us to choose relatively large dosage-intervals. For that reason the result of only one cat heart is expressed in figure Ic.

Discussion

The action of ouabain at extremely low concentrations on guinea-pig and cat heart contractility was characterized by a distinct, bell-shaped positive inotropic effect. This effect disappeared at higher concentrations and reappeared at tenfold higher concentrations of the drug. On rat heart, however, instead of a bell-shaped effect a flat sigmoid course of the logdose-response curve was observed in the lower concentration area. At the highest concentrations of ouabain the inotropic effects on rat and on guinea-pig hearts were in full agreement with data available from literature (Ito et al., 1970; Fricke et al., 1975). From these results, we concluded that the positive inotropic effect of ouabain on mammalian heart is biphasic in character and has to be regarded as the result of two separate mechanisms of action.

Our hypothesis to explain these two separate positive inotropic actions of ouabain is based on four lines of evidence extracted from the literature; (1) the striking similarity in in vitro as well as in vivo effects of digitalis glycosides and extracellular Ca^{2+} (Loewie, 1917); (2) a digitalis-induced stimulation of the sarcolemmal Na^+/K^+-pump system at relatively low drug concentrations (Lee and Klaus, 1971; Pitts and Askari, 1971; Blood, 1975; Cohen et al., 1976; Godfraind and Ghysel-Burton, 1977) and an inhibition of this enzyme system at higher concentrations (Dunham and Glynn, 1961; Repke, 1964; Akera and Brody, 1977); (3) a digitalis-induced increase in the availability of reversibly-bound sarcolemmal Ca which is thought to be involved in the control of cardiac contractility (Lüllmann and Holland, 1962; Nayler, 1973; Klaus and Krebs, 1974; Lüllmann and Peters, 1974; Bailey, 1977; Bentfeld et al., 1977; Sheridan, 1978; Akera et al., 1979; Halliday and Harding, 1979); and (4) the existence of at least two different receptor types for digitalis glycosides with clearly different receptor binding affinities (Baker and Willis, 1972; Lüllmann and Ravens, 1973; Godfraind, 1975; Heller and Beck, 1978; Ghysel-Burton and Godfraind, 1979; La Bella, 1979; De Pover and Godfraind, 1979). A scheme for the mechanism of action of ouabain is given in figure II. At low concentrations, ouabain may interact with receptor-I (or high-affinity binding sites for ouabain). This receptor I-complex may lead to conformational changes in sarcolemmal glycoproteins and adjacent phospholipid structures and via this process to a specific increment in the availability of sarcolemmal-bound calcium. Upon each membrane-depolarization more sarcolemmal-Ca may be released from or move across the cell membrane into the cytoplasm and the subsequent rise in intracellular free Ca^{2+} concentration may induce the "first" positive inotropic effect.

The "second" positive inotropic effect, observed at higher concentrations of ouabain may be regarded as the ultimate result of an occupation of receptor-II (or low-affinity binding sites). The drug-receptor-II-complex obtained now may act as the initial step in a process leading to a Ca_{SL}-mediated inhibition of the Na^+/K^+-pump (Gervais et al., 1977) and via this step indirectly to an increase in myocardial contractility (see for an extensive review, Akera and Brody, 1977).

The fact that the "first" positive inotropic effect of ouabain on guinea-pig and cat heart disappeared with increasing drug concentrations implicated that the interaction of ouabain

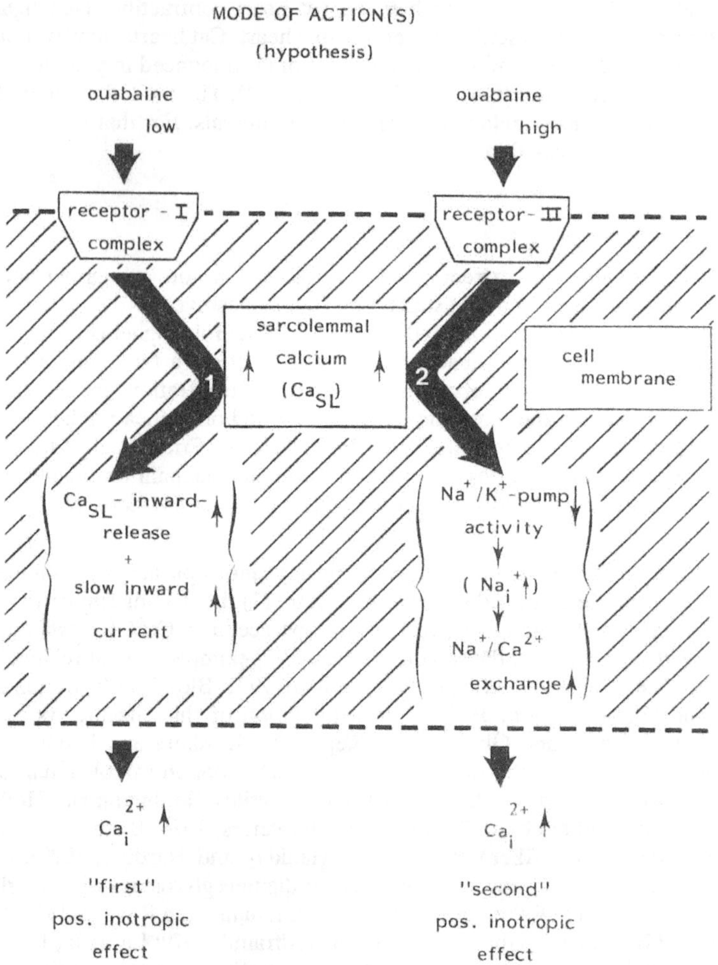

Fig. II. Hypothetical scheme describing the biphasic positive inotropic action of ouabain.

with receptor-I had to be very complex. It was assumed that ouabain is able to form more than one type of complex with these binding sites and that only one of these complexes is pharmacologically active. If this assumption is true, the ouabain molecule itself has to possess at least two chemically active binding sites (Gero, 1969; two-point attachment). A mathematical description of the dose-response relationship is given in the next equation:

$$E^{I+II} = \frac{\omega E^{I}_{max}}{K_1/(ouab) + K_2(ouab) + K_3 + 1} + \frac{E^{II}_{max}(ouab)}{K_{II} + (ouab)}$$

E^{I+II}: overall contractile response; (ouab): the corresponding concentration of ouabain; E^{I}_{max} and E^{II}_{max}: maximal responses obtainable with each receptor type; K_1, K_2 and K_3: compound equilibrium (dissociation-) constants belonging to the three different ouabain-receptor-I-interactions; K_{II}: dissociation constant for receptor-II and ω proportionality constant.

Although we found clear differences in species sensitivity to ouabain and in the character of the contractile responses to ouabain obtained from hearts of the different species used, it was possible to fit* the experimental results obtained with rat (fig. Ia), guinea-pig (fig. Ib) and cat heart (fig. Ic) properly with this mathematical equation (see computer-drawn lines in fig. Ia-c and compare them with the experimental data). In this context, it has to be remarked that studies on rat heart function often yield results which differ clearly from those obtained with other mammalian species. However, Forester and Mainwood (1974) not only found a normal force-frequency relationship for rat heart when extracellular Ca^{2+} was lowered, but also an increased sensitivity to ouabain. The amount of calcium bound to the cardiac sarcolemma generally is considered to be closely dependent upon the prevailing extracellular Ca^{2+}-concentration.

In conclusion, the observed biphasic positive inotropic action of ouabain on isolated hearts of three different mammalian species strongly supports the existence of two different mechanisms of action of ouabain. The proposed possibility to express both inotropic effects within one single mathematical equation which is suitable for all three species suggest an interdependency between both mechanisms of action of ouabain. In our opinion the binding characteristics of calcium ions to the sarcolemmal surface structures are an important factor in both mechanisms of action of ouabain.

Appendix

Suppose there are two different types of receptor for ouabain. At low concentrations the effect of ouabain, E^I, is regarded as the ultimate result of an occupation of high-affinity binding sites, R^I. The bell-shaped part (guinea-pig and cat heart) of the dose-response curve agrees well with the two-point attachment theory of Gero (1968). Translation of his mathematical formulation to our case gives the following equation

$$E^I = \frac{\alpha(R^I)t}{K_1/(ouab) + K_2(ouab) + K_3 + 1} \tag{2}$$

where E^I is the effect of ouabain due to interaction with R^I; α is the intrinsic activity; $(R^I)_t$ is the total number of R^I; K_1, K_2 and K_3 are equilibrium constants of ouabain and the different R^I-complexes possible; (ouab) is the concentration of ouabain resulting in E^I. Differentiation of E^I with respect to (ouab) in eq. 2 gives

$$\alpha(R^I)_t = 2\sqrt{(K_1/K_2} + K_3 + 1 \quad E^I_{max} \tag{3}$$

or

$$\alpha(R^I)_t = \omega E^I_{max} \tag{4}$$

in which the constant ω represents the reciprocal value of the fraction of $(R^I)_t$ which is equal to the total number of pharmacologically active ouabain-R^I-complexes.
Substitution of eq. (3) into eq. (2) gives

*A computer listing of the curve-fitting procedure is available on request from the authors.

$$E^{I} = \frac{\omega E^{I}_{max}}{K_1/(ouab) + K_2(ouab) + K_3 + 1} \tag{5}$$

The shape of the second part of the dose-response curves (all three species used) of ouabain made us to suppose that the second receptor type, R^{II} (or low-affinity binding sites), is saturable in character. The mathematical formulation of such an ouabain-R^{II}-interaction will be as given in eq. (5) according to Ariëns (1956).

$$E^{II} = \frac{E^{II}_{max}\,(ouab)}{k_{II} + (ouab)} \tag{6}$$

(k_{II} is the dissociation constant of the ouabain-R^{II}-complex)

From our model describing the mode of action of ouabain it appeared that both effects are due to an increase in the free intracellular Ca^{2+} concentration. For this reason we suppose additivity of both effects

$$E^{I+II} = E^{I} + E^{II} \tag{7}$$

and substitution of eq. (4) and (5) into eq. (6) will give

$$E^{I+II} = \frac{\omega E^{I}_{max}}{K_1/(ouab) + K_2(ouab) + K_3 + 1} + \frac{E^{II}_{max}(ouab)}{k_{II} + (ouab)} \tag{8}$$

in which E^{I+II} is the overall-effect of ouabain regardless of which receptor type is activated.

References

1. Akera T, Brody TM (1977) The role of Na^{+},K^{+}-ATPase in the inotropic action of digitalis. Pharmacol Rev 29:187–220
2. Akera T, Hirai M, Oka T (1979) Sodium ions and the development of the inotropic action of ouabain in guinea-pig heart. Eur J Pharmacol 60:189–198
3. Bailey LE (1977) Changes in myocardial calcium and E-C coupling associated with failure and ouabain treatment. Arch Int Pharmacodyn 226:118–131
4. Baker PF, Willis JS (1972) Binding of the cardiac glycoside ouabain to intact cells. J Physiol 224:441–462
5. Bentfeld M, Lüllmann H, Peters T, Proppe D (1977) Interdependence of ion transport and the action of ouabain in heart muscle. Br J Pharmacol 61:19–27
6. Blood BE (1975) The influence of low doses of ouabain and potassium ions on sheep Purkinje fibre contractility. J Physiol 251:69P
7. Cohen I, Daut J, Noble D (1976) An analysis of the actions of low concentrations of ouabain on membrane currents in Purkinje fibres. J Physiol 260:75–103
8. De Pover A, Godfraind T (1979) Interaction of ouabain with (Na^{+}+K^{+})-ATPase from human heart and from guinea-pig heart. Biochem Pharmacol 28:3051–3056
9. Dunham ET, Glynn IM (1961) Adenosinetriphophatase activity and the active movements of alkali metal ions. J Physiol 156:274–293
10. Forester GV, Mainwood GW (1974) Interval dependent inotropic effects in the rat myocardium and the effect of calcium. Pflügers Arch 352:189–196
11. Fricke N, Hollborn N, Klaus W (1975) Inotropic action, myocardial uptake and subcellular distribution of ouabain, digoxin and digitoxin in isolated rat hearts. Naunyn-Schmiedeberg's Arch Pharmacol 228:195–214
12. Gero A Physico-chemical aspects of drug actions. In: Third Int Pharmacol Meeting Vol 7 ed EJ Ariens pp 261–269. New York/Pergamon Press 1968

13. Gervais A, Lane LK, Anner BM, Lindenmayer GE, Schwartz A (1977) A possible molecular mechanism of the action of digitalis. Ouabain action on calcium binding to sites associated with a purified sodium-potassium-activated adenosine triphosphatase from kidney. Circulation Res 40:8–14
14. Ghysel-Burton J, Godfraind T (1979) Stimulation and inhibition of the sodium pump by cardioactive steroids in relation to their binding sites and their inotropic effect on guinea-pig isolated atria. Br J Pharmacol 66:175–184
15. Godfraind T (1975) Cardiac glycoside receptors in the heart. Biochem Pharmacol 24:823–827
16. Godfraind T, Ghysel-Burton J (1977) Binding sites related to ouabain-induced stimulation or inhibition of the sodium pump. Nature 265:165–166
17. Halliday J, Harding SE (1979) Modification of the negative inotropic effect of lanthanum by ouabain and some other positive inotropic agents. Br J Pharmacol 66:85P
18. Heller M, Beck S (1978) Interactions of cardiac glycosides with cells and membranes. Properties and structural aspects of two receptor sites for ouabain in erythrocytes. Biochim Biophys Acta 514:332–347
19. Ito M, Hollander PB, Marks BH, Dutta S (1970) The effect of six cardiac glycosides on the transmembrane potential and contractile characteristics of the right ventricle of guinea pigs. J Pharmacol Exp Ther 172:188–195
20. Klaus W, Krebs R (1974) Kinetische Analyse der Calcium-Kompartimente im Meerschweinchenherzen unter Kontrollbedingungen und Strophanthineinwirkung. Naunyn-Schmiedeberg's Arch Pharmacol 283:277–292
21. La Bella FS, Bihler I, Kim RS (1979) Progesterone derivative binds to cardiac ouabain receptor and shows dissociation between sodium pump inhibition and increased contractile force. Nature 278:571–573
22. Lee KS, Klaus W (1971) The subcellular basis for the mechanism of inotropic action of cardiac glycosides. Pharmacol Rev 23:194–261
23. Loewie von O (1917) Über den Zusammenhang zwischen Digitalis- und Kalziumwirkung. Arch Exp Pathol Pharmacol 82:131–158
24. Lüllmann H, Holland W (1962) Influence of ouabain on an exchangeable calcium fraction, contractile force and resting tension of guinea-pig atria. J Pharmacol Exp Ther 137:186–192
25. Lüllmann H, Ravens U (1973) The time courses of the changes in contractile force and in transmembrane potentials induced by cardiac glycosides in guinea-pig papillary muscle. Br J Pharmacol 49:377–390
26. Lüllmann H, Peters T Cardiac glycosides and contractility. In: Adv Cardiol Vol 12: The myocardium, pp 174–182. Basel: Karger 1974
27. Nayler WG (1973) An effect of ouabain on the superficially-located stores of calcium in cardiac muscle cells. J Mol Cell Cardiol 5:101–110
28. Okita GT (1977) Dissociation of Na^+,K^+-ATPase inhibition from digitalis inotropy. Fed Proc 36:2225–2230
29. Peters T, Raben R-H, Wassermann O (1974) Evidence for a dissociation between positive inotropic effect and inhibition of the $(Na^+ + K^+)$-ATPase by ouabain, cassaine and their alkylating derivatives. Eur J Pharmacol 26:166–174
30. Pitts BJ, Askari A (1971) Stimulation of the phosphatase activity of (Na^+,K^+)-ATPase preparations by ouabain. Biochim Biophys Acta 225:388–391
31. Repke K (1964) Über den biochemischen Wirkungsmodus von Digitalis. Klin Wschr 42:157–165
32. Sheridan DJ (1978) Effects of ouabain on contraction and superficially bound calcium in neonatal and adult cardiac muscles. J Mol Cell Cardiol 10:1123–1129

Authors' address:

Dr. J. M. Koomen, Faculty of Pharmacy, Department of Pharmacology, State University of Utrecht, Catharijnesingel 60, 3511 GH Utrecht (The Netherlands)

Digitalis receptors affinity labelling and relation with positive inotropic and cardiotoxic effects

M. Lazdunski, T. Kazazoglou, J. F. Renaud, and B. Rossi

Centre de Biochimie, Centre National de la Recherche Scientifique, Faculté des Sciences, Nice Cedex (France)

Summary

Affinity labelling of the digitalis receptor has indicated that it is situated on the N-terminal part of the α-subunit of the (Na^+,K^+)ATPase.

Biochemical and pharmacological properties of the (Na^+,K^+)ATPase studied on intact chick embryonic hearts and under heart cell culture conditions have indicated the existence of two families of ouabain binding sites *i.e.*: a low affinity binding sites with a dissociation constant (K_d) of 2–6 μM for the ouabain-receptor complex and a high affinity binding site with a K_d of 26–48 nM. High and low affinity sites also are present at all embryonic stages studied. Inhibition of $^{86}Rb^+$ uptake in cultured cardiac cells and increase in intracellular Na^+ concentration, due to (Na^+,K^+)ATPase blockade, occur in an ouabain concentration range corresponding to the saturation of the low affinity ouabain site. Ouabain stimulated $^{45}Ca^{2+}$ uptake increases in parallel with the increase in the intracellular Na^+ concentration. It is suppressed in Na^+ free medium or when Na^+ is replaced by Li^+ suggesting that the increase is due to the indirect activation of the Na^+/Ca^{2+} exchange system in the plasma membrane. Dose-response curves for the inotropic effects of ouabain on papillary muscle and on ventricular cells in culture indicate the development of the cardiotonic properties is parallel to the saturation of the low affinity binding site for ouabain. Therefore, inhibition of the cardiac (Na^+,K^+)ATPase corresponding to low affinity ouabain binding sites seems to be responsible for both the cardiotonic and cardiotoxic effects of the drug.

Key words: affinity labelling, digitalis receptor, heart, Na^+/Ca^{2+} exchange system, inotropy

Introduction

Digitalis compounds exert a positive inotropic effect on cardiac muscle. The effects of these cardiotonic steroids have been extensively studied but there is no general agreement on the mechanism by which they increase the strength of contraction. A number of investigators have suggested that the positive inotropic effect is a consequence of a transient increase in intracellular Na^+ concentration caused by a partial inhibition of the (Na^+,K^+)ATPase; the accumulation of Na^+ then causes an increase in intracellular Ca^{2+} by the Na^+/Ca^{2+} exchange system (1–15). However, there are also a number of investigators who argue that (Na^+,K^+)ATPase is not the pharmacological receptor or at least not the only pharmacological receptor for the inotropic effect of digitalis compounds (10, 16–22). The problem is now complicated by the fact that a number of recent publications have reported that there exist at least two families of ouabain binding sites in cardiac tissue (17, 23–33). It is not yet entirely clear whether these two families of sites correspond to two families of (Na^+,K^+)ATPases or to two different types of ouabain receptors corresponding to two different types of physiological activities. Affinity labelling of the digitalis receptor has indicated that it is situated on the N-terminal part of the α-subunit of the (Na^+,K^+)ATPase (34–37).

(Na^+,K^+)ATPase: sodium and potassium activated adenosine triphosphatase;

Affinity labelling of the digitalis receptor

A series of affinity labels for the identification of the molecular nature of the digitalis binding site have been recently developed (34–37). Some of these derivatives which have been most recently made and used in this laboratory are presented in Fig. 1 together with their mechanism (or probable mechanism) of action. All these derivatives which covalently associate with the digitalis receptor only incorporate in the α-chain (Mr ≊ 100,000) of the (Na^+,K^+)ATPase. A precise localisation of the peptide which contains the digitalis binding site has been recently established (Fig. 2).

Ouabain receptors in chick cardiac cells in culture and their relationship with (Na^+,K^+)ATPase inhibition, Ca^{2+} entry and contractile effects.

Results presented in Fig. 3 demonstrate that there are at least two families of binding sites of different affinity for ouabain in chick embryonic heart cells. Low affinity binding sites were identified by $[^3H]$ ouabain binding experiments on heart cell homogenates using direct equilibrium binding. The dissociation constant of the $[^3H]$ ouabain-receptor complex calculated from equilibrium binding is between 2 μM and 4 μM in the different chick heart preparations studied. Low affinity binding sites for ouabain are at a high level of 4.8 pmol/mg of protein in heart homogenate of 18-day-old chick embryos.

A second class of binding sites for $[^3H]$ ouabain is of high affinity corresponding to a dissociation constant value for the ouabain-receptor complex of 26 nM in 18-day-old chick embryonic heart homogenate. This value is about 100 times lower than the dissociation constant of the ouabain-receptor complex found for the low affinity binding sites. The amount of high affinity ouabain binding site is 0.6 pmol/mg of protein in heart homogenate from 18-day-old chick embryos and is about 10 times lower than the amount of low affinity binding sites. The binding characteristics of high and low affinities binding sites for ouabain in heart cells cultured as monolayers and as aggregates are K_d, 33 ± 6 nM and 3.9 ± 0.4 μM, and B_{Max} of 1.2 ± 0.2 pmol/mg of protein and 11.8 ± 0.8 pmol/mg of protein for the high and low affinity binding sites respectively. These values are not very different from the binding characteristics found in the homogenate of intact ventricles taken at the same age of *in ovo* development (40). The maximal binding capacities for ouabain correspond to values of 1.5×10^5 and 1.4×10^6 ouabain binding sites per cell for high and low affinity binding sites respectively.

High and low affinity binding sites for ouabain are already present at the youngest embryonic stage studied, *i.e.*: day 5 of *in ovo* development (40). During development *in ovo* the number of high affinity binding site gradually decreases from 1.3 pmol/mg protein at day 5 to 0.4 pmol/mg of protein at day 14 of development *in ovo* to stay nearly stable from 14 to 20 days. Conversely the number of low affinity binding sites is essentially invariant at a value of 6.4 ± 0.4 pmol/mg of protein between 5–20 days of development. Dissociation constants determined for the ouabain-receptor complex remain essentially invariant at all stages of development at a value of 41 ± 7 nM and 3.0 ± 0.3 μM for high and low affinities binding sites respectively.

A possible explanation for the existence of the small population of high affinity binding sites for ouabain in cardiac cells could be that these sites belong to presynaptic nervous components. However such an interpretation is unlikely for the following reasons: (i) During the course of embryonic development the number of high affinity binding sites decreases from 1.3 to 0.4 pmol/mg of protein, when innervation in ventricles becomes more extensive; (ii) When cardiac cells are grown in monolayers and in aggregate culture in the absence of nervous influence, they present about the same number of high affinity binding sites for ouabain as the intact heart taken at the same age of *in ovo* development (40).

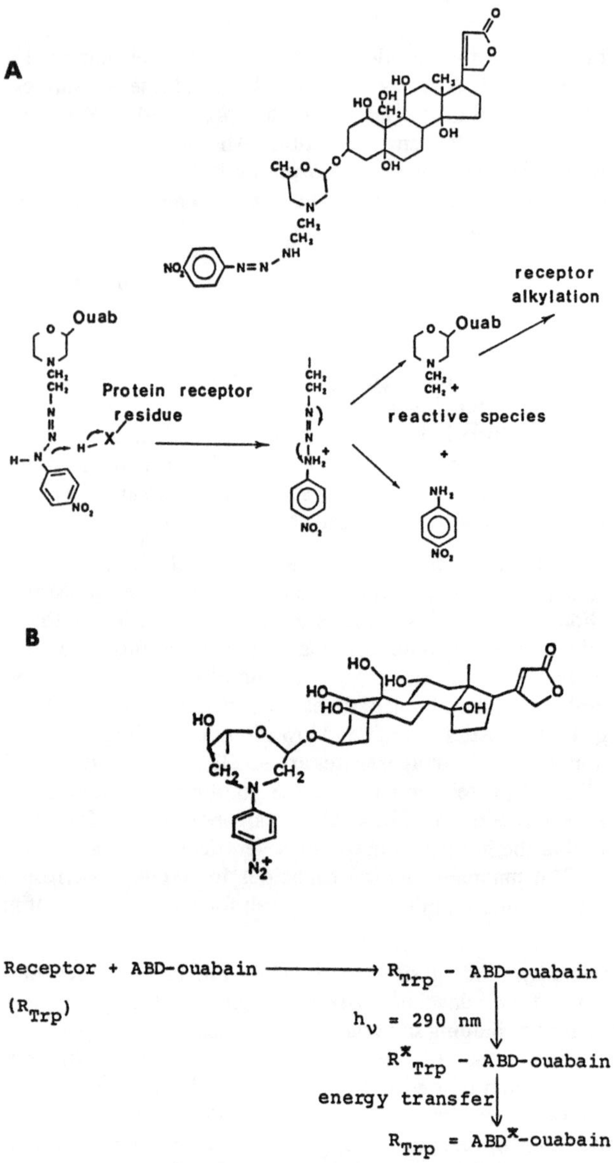

Fig. 1. *A. p-Nitrophenyltriazene ouabain (NPT-ouabain) is an alkylating modifier of the digitalis receptor.* The alkylation reaction involves a proton transfer from the receptor protein.
B. Aryldiazonium ouabain (ABD-ouabain) is a photoactivable reagent. It differs from other photoactivable derivatives of ouabain which have been already used by the fact that it is possible with that derivative to photoactivate selectively the molecule of reagent which is specifically bound to the digitalis receptor (and not the free molecules). This activation involves energy transfer through the excitation of tryptophan residues of the receptor protein.

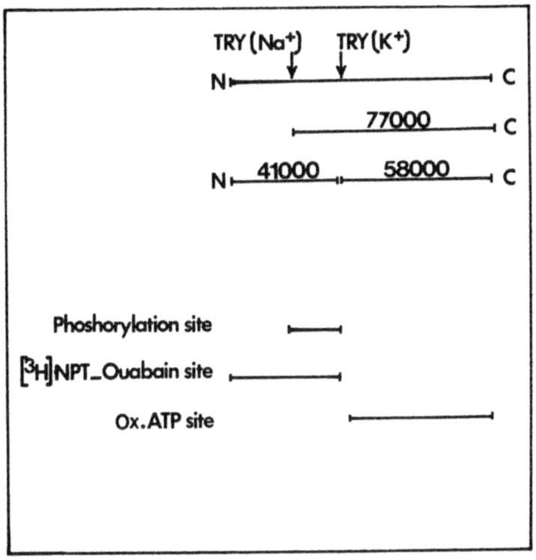

Fig. 2. *The mapping of the digitalis binding sites in the α-subunit sequence.* Positions of the primary tryptic cleavages (TRY) in the presence of K^+ or of Na^+ and N-terminal (N) and C-terminal residues (C) (38). The localization of the digitalis binding site has been made with NPT ouabain (36). Identical results have been obtained with ABD ouabain (37). The phosphorylation site (39) and the site for ATP labelled with oxidized ATP (ox-ATP) (39) are indicated for comparison.

The ouabain-sensitive $^{86}Rb^+$ uptake catalyzed by the (Na^+,K^+)ATPase is inhibited by ouabain in the same range of ouabain concentrations that is required to saturate the low affinity ouabain binding site in experiments with heart cells cultured as monolayers. No indication of inhibition of $^{86}Rb^+$ uptake was found in the ouabain concentration range corresponding to the high affinity binding sites (Fig. 4A), although we cannot completely eliminate the possibility that the $^{86}Rb^+$ flux component corresponding to high affinity ouabain binding sites is so small compared to that of the low affinity ouabain binding sites that it has not been detected. However, high affinity ouabain binding sites could well correspond to a physiologically non-functional (Na^+,K^+)ATPase.

The dose-response curve for the ouabain effect on the internal Na^+ concentration (Fig. 4B) shows that the half-maximum effect is observed at 2 μM ouabain, a value near that found for the half-maximum effect of ouabain on $^{86}Rb^+$ influx. In the absence of ouabain, the internal Na^+ concentration is 16 mM and it increases to 35 mM at saturating ouabain concentrations. The most plausible explanation for this maximal value of 32 to 36 mM, instead of a value for the internal Na^+ concentration near that of the external Na^+ concentration, is that there exists another route or routes for Na^+ efflux distinct from the (Na^+,K^+)ATPase system. The most obvious candidate is the Na^+/Ca^{2+} exchange system which would couple Na^+ efflux to Ca^{2+} entry. Such a system has indeed been identified in cell membranes of various tissues (11, 43–46). The internal Na^+ dependence of the initial rate of Ca^{2+} entry is very cooperative with a Hill coefficient of about 3 (43) and a half-maximum effect near 30 mM of internal Na^+. Thus, because of the very cooperative effect, a small increase of intracellular Na^+ concentration from the physiological concentration will produce a large increase in Ca^{2+} uptake.

Ouabain considerably stimulates the initial rate of $^{45}Ca^{2+}$ entry as shown in Fig. 4C. The concentration dependence of ouabain action indicates a half-maximum effect of 3 μM. Table 1 shows that there is an excellent correspondence between half-maximum effects of ouabain on $^{86}Rb^+$ uptake, internal Na^+ concentration, and initial rates of Ca^{2+} uptake. All these effects

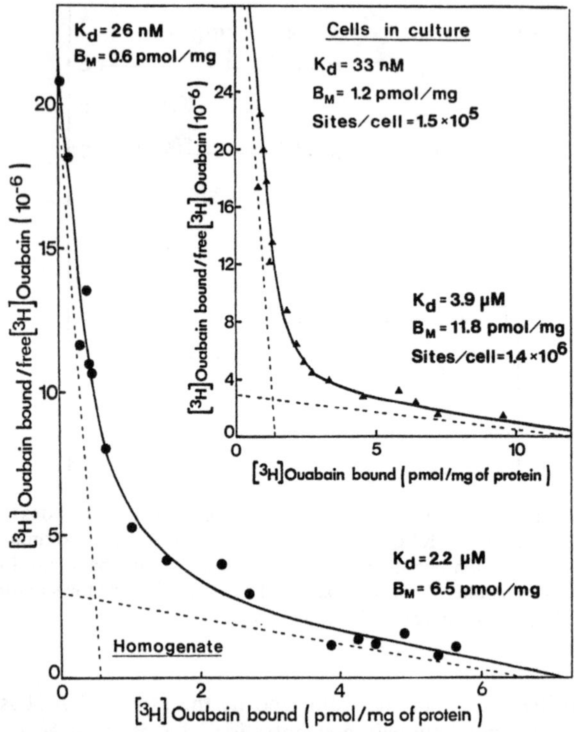

Fig. 3. *Binding of [^{3}H] ouabain to embryonic heart homogenates and intact embryonic heart cells cultured as monolayers* (41). Main panel: Scatchard plot for the specific binding of [^{3}H] ouabain to 18-day-old embryonic heart homogenate (●) was measured as previously described (40). Specific binding compared to total binding was 89 % and 75 % at K_d = 26 nM and K_d = 2.2 μM respectively. Inset: Scatchard plots indicate the existence of both high and low affinity binding sites for ouabain in intact heart cells (▲). Curvilinear plots were fitted according to a two-site model assuming the existence of two independent classes of ouabain-binding sites (42). Dotted line corresponding to the family of high and low affinity sites were obtained using regression analysis.

Table 1. Relationship between low affinity binding sites for ouabain and the effect of the drug on ^{86}Rb influx, intracellular Na^+, $^{45}Ca^{2+}$ uptake and contraction in chick heart

	dissociation constants and half-maximum effects
[^{3}H] ouabain binding[1]	2–4 μM
$^{86}Rb^+$ flux	5.6 μM
Intracellular Na^+ content	2 μM
$^{45}Ca^{2+}$ influx	3 μM
Inotropic effects[2]	1–2 μM

[1]Values obtained from equilibrium binding.
[2]Values obtained with papillary muscle and aggregates of ventricular cells

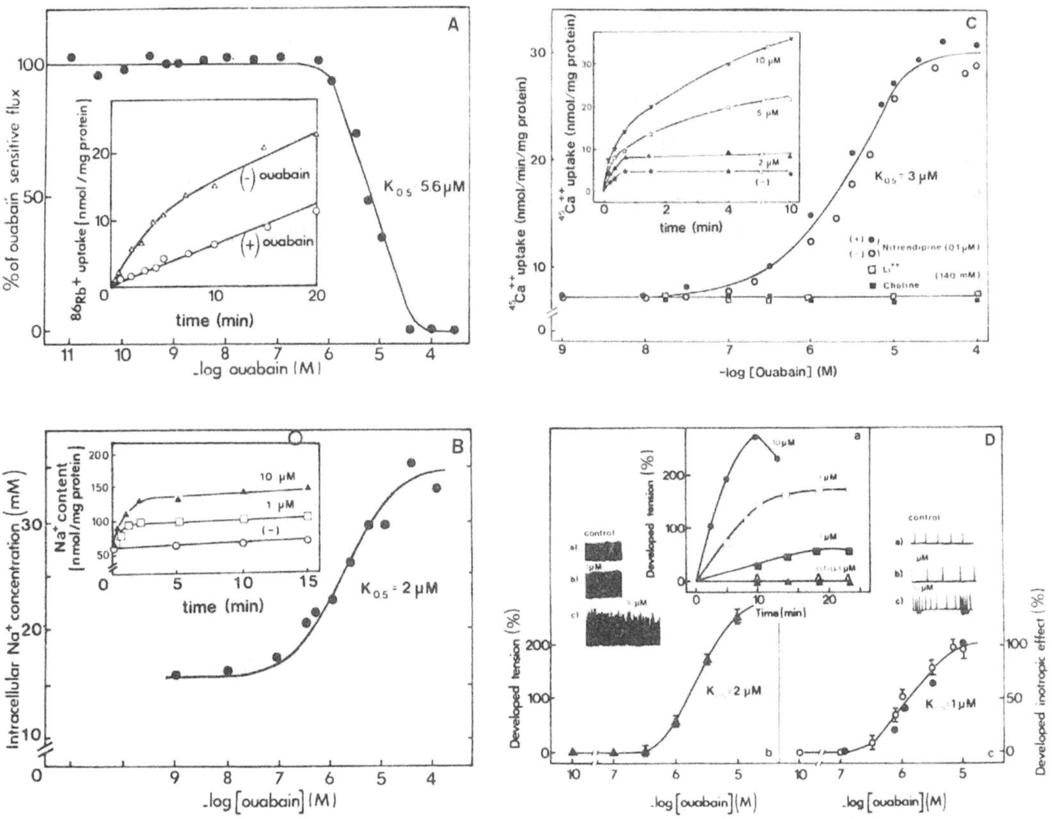

Fig. 4. The action of ouabain on the rates of $^{86}Rb^+$ uptake (A) on the intracellular Na^+ concentration (B) and on the rates of $^{45}Ca^{2+}$ uptake (C) by 11-day-old chick embryonic heart cells cultured as monolayers. *Inset A:* Time course of $^{86}Rb^+$ uptake in the presence (○) or absence (△) of 0.1 mM ouabain. *Main panel A:* Dose-response curve for the inhibition by ouabain of the initial rate of $^{86}Rb^+$ uptake (●). *Inset B:* Kinetics of Na^+ accumulation measured in the absence and presence of different ouabain concentrations. *Main panel B:* Effect of increasing ouabain concentrations in equilibrium conditions on the internal Na^+ cell content (●). *Inset C:* Time course of $^{45}Ca^{2+}$ uptake measured in the absence and presence of different ouabain concentrations. *Main panel C:* Effect of increasing ouabain concentrations on the initial rates of $^{45}Ca^{2+}$ uptake in the absence (○) or presence of 0.1 μM nitrendipine (●) and after replacement of the external Na^+ by Li^+ (□) and choline (■). *Panel D* shows (a) the time course of development of the positive inotropic action of varying ouabain concentrations. Ouabain dose-response curve (b) on development tension of stimulated isolated chick ventricular muscle and (c) on spontaneously beating cells cultured in form aggregate. *Inset b and c:* Recording of the contraction for isolated ventricular muscles and aggregates respectively.

are related to the saturation of the low affinity ouabain binding site. The close relationship which exists between the effects of ouabain on internal Na^+ concentration and the effects of ouabain on initial rates of Ca^{2+} entry suggests that Ca^{2+} entry is due to the operation of the Na^+/Ca^{2+} exchange system. This conclusion is supported by two observations (i) the ouabain stimulated Ca^{2+} flux occurs even in the presence of blockers of voltage-dependent Ca^{2+} channels like nitrendipine, eliminating the possibility of a $^{45}Ca^{2+}$ entry through voltage-dependent Ca^{2+} channels which would be activated by a membrane depolarization produced by ouabain, (ii) the ouabain-stimulated Ca^{2+} flux is inhibited by replacement of Na^+ in the external medium by Li^+ or choline. Li^+ is well known to accumulate in cells and to block the Na^+/Ca^{2+} exchange system (47–49).

Dose-response curves for the inotropic effect of ouabain measured by different techniques (50–51) using papillary muscle or cardiac cells in culture (Fig. 4D) are also closely similar to dose-response curves describing the effect of ouabain on $^{86}Rb^+$ influx, internal Na^+ accumulation, $^{45}Ca^{2+}$ influx and lengthening of the action potential duration (Fig. 4A-B-C-D and Table 1). Therefore, it seems that the inotropic effect of the digitalis compound is due to the inhibition of the (Na^+,K^+) ATPase activity corresponding to the low affinity ouabain binding site, through an activation of the Na^+/Ca^{2+} exchange system in the plasma membrane and the subsequent increase of the intracellular Na^+ concentration. When the enzyme is partially inhibited an inotropic effect is found, and extensive inhibition (>50%) results in arrhythmia. The increase in intracellular Na^+ concentration could of course also release Ca^{2+} from intracellular stores and particularly from mitochondria (52–53), but this aspect of the action of ouabain has not been studied here.

In rat myocardium, high (K_d = 3.9 nM) and low (K_d = 1 μM) affinity binding sites for ouabain have also been found by us and others (29, 30, 54–55). In this system, only the low affinity sites seem to be linked to sodium pump inhibition (32, 54–55) and Na^+/Ca^{2+} exchange system alteration (55) as reported here for chick hearts, whereas the positive inotropic effects of the rat myocardium due to low concentrations of ouabain (high affinity sites) do not seem to be linked to (Na^+,K^+) pump inhibition (30, 32, 55) and to Na^+–Ca^{++} exchange activation (55). In guinea pig heart it has also been proposed that there are high and low affinity binding sites for ouabain and that inotropic action cannot be entirely due to the glycoside-evoked inhibition of the (Na^+,K^+)ATPase (20, 56). The physiological role of the high affinity binding sites and the molecular differences between high and low affinities ouabain binding sites remain to be discovered.

It is of interest to remark that the existence of different classes of ouabain sites is not a property which is unique to cardiac cells. High (K_d = 50–60 nM) and low (K_d = 20–40 μM) affinity binding sites have also been found in preadipocyte cell lines (57) and in this case only the second class of low affinity binding sites is functional for $^{86}Rb^+$ transport. High and low affinity binding sites for ouabain has also been found in ouabain resistant mutants of a canine kidney cell line, MDCK, but in this case the levels of high and low affinity binding sites are equivalent (58) and both families of ouabain sites correspond to functional populations of (Na^+,K^+)ATPases. Results obtained with ouabain resistant mutants (58) strongly suggest that the mammalian genome contains a family of genes for the (Na^+,K^+)ATPase. Expression of a particular gene in the family would then be regulated according to environmental or developmental conditions (58). The high affinity site for ouabain, in embryonic chick cardiac cells, for which there is no evident physiological function may be expressed only after birth or after heart innervation becomes functional.

Acknowledgments

We thank Dr. M. P. Goeldner and Dr. Ph. Lapalus for many fruitful discussions. This work was supported by the Centre National de la Recherche Scientifique, The Institut National de la Santé et de la Recherche Médicale (PRC 131006) and the Fondation pour la Recherche Médicale.

References

1. Ku D, Akera T, Pew CL, Brody TM (1974) Naunyn-Schmiedeberg's Arch Pharmacol 285:185–200
2. Reuter H (1974) Circ Res 34:599–605
3. Schwartz A, Lindenmayer GE, Allen JC (1975) Pharmacol Rev 27:3–134
4. Akera T, Brody TM (1977) Pharmacol Rev 29:187–220
5. Gelbart A, Goldman RH (1977) Biochim Biophys Acta 481:689–694
6. Allen DG, Blinks JR (1978) Nature 273:509–513
7. Weingart R, Kass RS, Tsien RW (1978) Nature 273:389–301
8. Wood JM, Schwartz A (1978) J Mol Cell Cardiol 10:137–144
9. Biedert S, Barry WH, Smith TW (1979) J Gen Physiol 74:479–494
10. Noble D (1980) Cardiovas Res 14:495–514
11. Langer GA (1981) Biochem Pharmacol 30:3261–3264
12. Cohen CJ, Fozzard HA, Sheu SS (1982) Circ Res 50:651–662
13. Eisner DA, Lederer WJ (1982) Proc R Soc B 214:249–262
14. Sheu SS, Fozzard HA (1982) J Gen Physiol 80:325–351
15. Marban E, Tsien RW (1982) J Physiol 329:589–614
16. Okita GT, Ten Eick RE, Richardson F (1974) Ann N Y Acad Sci 242:658–670
17. Godfraind T, Ghysel-Burton J (1977) Nature 265:165–166
18. Okita GT (1977) Fed Proc 36:1115–2230
19. Michael L, Pitts BJR, Schwartz A (1978) Science 200:1287–1289
20. Godfraind T, Ghysel-Burton J (1980) Proc Natl Acad Sci 77:3067–3069
21. Rhee HM, Dutta S, Marks BH (1976) Eur J Pharmacol 37:141–153
22. Rhee HM, Huang WH, Askari A (1981) Eur J Pharmacol 70:273–278
23. Taniguchi K, Iida S (1972) Biophys Acta 288:98–102
24. Inagaki C, Lindenmayer GE, Schwartz A (1974) J Biol Chem 249:5135–5140
25. Hansen O (1976) Biochim Biophys Acta 433:383–392
26. Choi YR, Akera T (1977) Biochim Biophys Acta 481:648–659
27. Fricke U, Klaus W (1977) Br J Pharmacol 61:423–428
28. Van Alstyne E, Bartschat DK, Poe SL and Lindenmayer GE: Fed Proc 37:779
29. De Pover A, Godfraind, T (1979) Biochem Pharmacol 28:3051–3056
30. Erdmann E, Philipp G, Scholz H (1980) Biochem Pharmacol 29:3219–3229
31. Wellsmith NY, Lindenmayer GE (1980) Circ Res 47:710–720
32. Adams RJ, Schwartz A, Grupp G, Grupp I, Lee SW, Wallick ET, Powell T, Twist VW, Gathiram P (1982) Nature 296:167–169
33. Mansier P, Lelievre LG (1983) Nature 300:535–537
34. Forbush B, Kaplan JH, Hoffman JF (1978) Biochemistry 17:3667–3675
35. Rogers TB, Lazdunski M (1979) Biochemistry 18:135–140
36. Rossi B, Vuillleumier P, Gache C, Balerna M, Lazdunski M (1980) J Biol Chem 255:9936–9941
37. Goeldner MP, Hirth CG, Rossi B, Ponzio G, Lazdunski M (1983) Biochemistry 22:4685–4690
38. Castro J, Farley RA (1979) J Biol Chem 254:2221–2228
39. Ponzio G, Rossi B, Lazdunski M (1983) J Biol Chem 258:8799–8805
40. Kazazoglou T, Renaud JF, Rossi B, Lazdunski M (1983) J Biol Chem 258:12163–12170
41. Renaud JF (1980) Biol Cell 37:97–104
42. Fehlmann M, Morin O, Kitabgi P, Freychet P (1981) Endocrinology 109:263–261
43. Goshima K, Wakabayashi S (1981) J Mol Cell Cardiol 13:489–509
44. Blaustein MP (1974) Rev Physiol Biochem Pharmacol 70:33–82
45. Sulakhe PV, St Louis PJ (1980) In "Progress in Biophysics and Molecular Biology" 35:135–195
46. Wakabayashi S, Goshima K (1981) Biochim Biophys Acta 642:158–172
47. Reuter H, Seitz N (1968) J Physiol (Lond) 195:451–470
48. Baker PF, Blaustein MP, Hodgkin AL, Steinhardt RA (1969) J Physiol (Lond) 200:431–458
49. Ponce-Hornos JE, Langer GA (1980) J Mol Cell Cardiol 12:1367–1382
50. Fayet G, Couraud F, Miranda F, Lissitzky S (1974) Eur J Pharmacol 87:165–174
51. Bordes M, Bernengo JC, Renaud JF (1983) Rev Sci Intr 54:1053–1058
52. Crompton M, Capano M, Carafoli E (1976) Eur J Biochem 69:453–462
53. Carafoli E (1979) FEBS Lett 104:1–5
54. Werdan K, Krawietz W, Erdmann E (1983) J Mol Cell Cardiol 8:abstract p 15

55. Godfraind T, Noël F, Finet M (1983) J Mol Cell Cardiol 8:abstract p 43
56. Godfraind T, Ghysel-Burton J, De Pover A (1982) Nature 299:824–826
57. Forest C, Ponzio G, Rossi B, Lazdunski M, Ailhaud G (1982) Biochem Biophys Res Commun 107:422–428
58. Soderberg K, Rossi B, Lazdunski M, Louvard D (1983) J Biol Chem 258:12300–12307

Authors' address:

Dr. M. Lazdunski, Centre de Biochimie. Centre National de la Recherche Scientifique, Faculté des Sciences, Parc Valrose, 06034 Nice Cedex (France)

Two ouabain binding sites in guinea pig heart Na^+–K^+–ATPase. Differentiation by sodium and erythrosin B

U. Fricke

Pharmakologisches Institut der Universität zu Köln, Köln (FRG)

Summary

^3H-ouabain binding to guinea pig heart NaK-ATPase resulted in two different cardiac glycoside binding sites: A high affinity, low capacity binding was obtained at a $K_D = 2.6 \times 10^{-7}$ mol/l (about 40% of the binding sites) whereas a low affinity, high capacity binding was established at a $K_D = 1.3 \times 10^{-6}$ mol/l (about 60% of the binding sites). Similar results were obtained when studying the effect of increasing Na^+-concentrations on ouabain binding: again two distinct processes involved in the Na^+/ouabain interaction could be demonstrated. Whereas one ouabain binding process was activated at rather low Na^+-concentrations ($K_{0.5} = 4.5$ mmol/l), the other ouabain binding process was predominant at high Na^+-concentrations only ($K_{0.5} = 69$ mmol/l). Comparing these data with the ouabain action on contractile force and with NaK-ATPase activity in guinea pig heart, the high affinity binding of ouabain seems to correlate with the inotropic action, whereas the low affinity ouabain binding is more related to NaK-ATPase inhibition.

To further discriminate the two cardiac glycoside binding sites operative in guinea pig heart muscle, erythrosin B, shown to be an inhibitor of the high affinity ouabain binding in this preparation, was applied to isolated guinea pig left atria in the presence of increasing ouabain concentrations. There was no change in the ouabain induced inotropy or toxicity by erythrosin B. These results could indicate that the low affinity ouabain binding is responsible for both inotropic and toxic actions in guinea pig heart. However, the functional significance of the high affinity ouabain binding would then remain obscure. Therefore, an alternate, and more plausible explanation for the lack of effect of erythrosin B on ouabain action in guinea pig atria would be an interaction of the dye with the ATP-site of the NaK-ATPase, which would suppose a cellular uptake of this drug, as yet not established.

Key words: ouabain binding, sodium, erythrosin B, functional significance, guinea pig heart

Introduction

In spite of a large body of publications and fascinating hypotheses concerning the mechanism of cardiac glycoside action, our present understanding of how digitalis works on the cellular level is still controversial (1, 12, 19, 22). Nevertheless, it is generally accepted that the cardiac (Na^+ + K^+)-activated adenosine-5′-triphosphatase (NaK-ATPase) is the primary binding site of these drugs (1, 4, 19, 22).

However, quantitation of the cardiac glycoside binding to the NaK-ATPase showed that, depending on the species and tissue studied, under different experimental conditions at least two binding sites could be revealed (6, 10, 11, 16, 23): a high affinity, low capacity binding of cardiac glycosides which in guinea pig and rat heart has been related to the positive inotropic action of these drugs (5, 6), and a low affinity, high capacity binding which seems to be more connected with the inhibition of the NaK-ATPase (5, 6). These results, however, are in disagreement with the respective experiments on more "digitalis-sensitive" species, e.g. cat, beef, dog or man, which resulted in only one ouabain binding site in cardiac NaK-ATPase (4).

As recently erythrosin B, an artificial food dye, has been reported to be a specific inhibitor of the high affinity ouabain binding in rat brain tissue (14, 23, 24), this drug might offer an opportunity to further discriminate the ouabain binding sites in heart muscle NaK-ATPase, and, when applied to the contracting heart, should give more information on the functional significance of the cardiac glycoside binding sites operative in guinea pig heart muscle.

Methods and Materials

Preparation of guinea pig heart NaK-ATPase

NaK-ATPase from guinea pig heart was freshly prepared before use as previously described (9). The final enzyme preparation was stored in an imidazole-HCl buffer (100 mmol/l imidazole-HCl, 1 mmol/l Na_2-EDTA, pH 7.4) and used for the experiments.

The NaK-ATPase activity was in the range of 5–8 µmol ATP hydrolyzed /hour/mg protein at 37 °C. About 80–90 % of the total activity was inhibited by 10^{-3} mol/l ouabain.

ATPase activity assay

Enzyme activities were determined at 37 °C in the presence of increasing concentrations of the drugs tested. Usually 10 µg of protein were preincubated for 10 min in 100 mmol/l imidazole-HCl buffer, pH 7.4, containing 5 mmol/l $MgCl_2$, 100 mmol/l NaCl, 5 mmol/l KCl and 1 mmol/l Na_2-EDTA. The reaction was started by the addition of ATP, the final concentration being 2 mmol/l. After 30 min, inorganic phosphate was determined by the methods of Eibl and Lands (3). Each assay was performed in duplicate. NaK-ATPase activity was calculated as the difference between total and Mg^{2+}, Na^+-dependent activity. The latter enzyme activity equalled the MgNaK-ATPase activity in the presence of 10^{-3} mmol/l ouabain.

^{3}H-ouabain binding

The binding studies were either performed as previously reported (10) or carried out according to the procedure described by Erdmann and Schoner (7, 8). Briefly, the experiments were either performed by incubation of the NaK-ATPase (about 0.3 mg of protein) with increasing concentrations of ^{3}H-ouabain (5–1000 mmol/l) in a medium of 5 mmol/l $MgCl_2$, various concentrations of NaCl (0–140 mmol/l), 1 mmol/l Na_2–EDTA, 100 mmol/l imidazole-HCl (pH 7.4) and 2 mmol/l Na_2-ATP at 37 °C for 30 min. Non-specific ^{3}H-ouabain binding was then estimated in the absence of ATP. The binding reaction was stopped after 30 min by immersion in an ice bath and subsequent centrifugation (40,000 g, 30 min, 0 °C). Bound ^{3}H-ouabain was determined in the resulting sediment by liquid scintillation counting (10).

The other series of experiments followed ouabain binding in the presence of 5 mmol/l $MgCl_2$, 3 mmol/l imidazole/PO_4^{3-} and increasing amounts of ^{3}H-ouabain (5–4,000 nmol/l) in 100 mmol/l imidazole-HCl buffer, pH 7.4. Non-specific binding was now determined in the presence of 10^{-3} mol/l unlabelled ouabain. After 30 min of incubation, bound ouabain was quantitated by rapid filtration (Whatman GF/C glass filter membranes) to separate free from membrane bound drug (7, 8).

All experiments were performed in duplicate assays.

Measurement of inotropic action

Inotropic action was evaluated on electrically stimulated right papillary muscles (60/min, 3 msec, 50 V) or left atria (120/min, 6 msec, 2 × threshold voltage), isolated from guinea pig hearts (guinea pigs of either sex, 200–250 g). Contractile force was measured isometrically by means of a force-displacement-transducer and recorded after amplification (Fleck, Mainz, FRG) on a thermorecorder (Hellige Servomed, Freiburg, FRG). The atria (resting tension: 1.0 g = 9.8 mN) and papillary muscles (resting tension: 0.5 g = 4.9 mN) were allowed to stabilize at 30 ° for about 60 min in an organ bath containing 10 ml of a modified Tyrode's solution (149 mmol/l Na^+, 5.4 mmol/l K^+, 0.9 mmol/l Ca^{2+}, 1.05 mmol/l Mg^{2+}, 144 mmol/l Cl^-, 11.9 mmol/l HCO_3^-, 0.42 mmol/l $H_2PO_4^-$ and 10.0 mmol/l glucose), which was equilibrated with 95 % O_2, 5 % CO_2 to give a pH of 7.4.

Drugs were dissolved in distilled water and usually added in a cumulative manner at 30 min intervals until toxic effects (contracture, arrhythmias) could be observed. The time intervals were chosen such as to allow a stable effect of drug action.

Miscellaneous

Protein concentrations were determined by the method of Lowry et al. (18) using Labtrol (Merz & Dade, München, FRG) as a standard. K_D values for direct binding studies with ^{3}H-ouabain were calculated from Hofstee-plots (15) and Scatchard-plots (20).

Indirect K_D values (for erythrosin B) were calculated according to Erdmann und Schoner (8).

The concentrations for half maximal inotropic response (ED_{50}) and half maximal inhibition of the NaK-ATPase (ID_{50}) were calculated from the individual concentration-effect-curves as proposed by Hafner et al. (13). All data were analysed by standard statistical methods (mean value and S.E. mean, regression analysis).

Materials

^{3}H-ouabain, specific activity 18 Ci/mmol, was purchased from New England Nuclear (Dreieich, FRG). Erythrosin B and Na_2-ATP were obtained from Serva (Heidelberg, FRG). All other chemicals were of analytical grade and were purchased from Merck (Darmstadt, FRG).

Results and discussion

Guinea pig myocardial NaK-ATPase incubated with increasing amounts of ^{3}H-ouabain (5–4,000 nmol/l) in the presence of Mg^{2+} and inorganic phosphate at 37 °C resulted in a saturable binding of ouabain, which, however, is not monophasic over the whole ouabain concentration range studied (fig. 1A). Analyzing these data according to Scatchard (20), the plot (fig. 1B) clearly demonstrates two populations of binding sites, one of which can be observed at low ouabain concentrations with a K_D-value of 2.6×10^{-7} mol/l, whereas the second binding site is obtained at rather high ouabain concentrations only, with a K_D-value of 1.3×10^{-6} mol/l. Respective maximum binding capacities (B_{max}) were calculated as 22 pmol ouabain/mg protein (high affinity, low capacity binding) and 37 pmol ouabain/mg protein (low affinity, high capacity binding). Similar different types of ouabain binding sites in guinea pig heart have also been demonstrated recently by Erdmann (5). The hitherto reported single class of ouabain binding sites in guinea pig heart muscle (2, 4), the K_D-value of which highly coincides with the K_D-value given above for the high affinity ouabain binding, therefore must result from a too narrow cardiac glycoside concentration range studied.

Two ouabain binding sites could also be established when the cardiac glycoside binding to guinea pig heart NaK-ATPase was studied in the presence of Mg^{2+}, ATP and increasing Na^+-concentrations (fig. 2A). Whereas ouabain binding in the absence of ATP was independent of the prevailing Na^+-concentrations, and therefore may be called "nonspecific", the ATP-dependent binding was highly dependent on the Na^+-concentration in the incubation medium. Within this ATP-dependent binding again two saturable ouabain binding components could be demonstrated, which became even more evident, when the data were replotted to the proposal of Hofstee (15) (fig. 2B). There is one population of ouabain binding sites which is activated at rather low Na^+-concentrations, with half maximal ouabain binding occurring at 4.5 mmol/l Na^+, whereas the other population of ouabain binding sites is predominant at high Na^+-concentrations with half maximal ouabain binding at 69 mmol/l Na^+. Comparable experiments on the influence of increasing Na^+-concentrations on the phosphorylation of guinea pig heart NaK-ATPase by ^{32}P-ATP (10), which resulted in one phosphorylation reaction with a Na^+-concentration for half maximum phosphorylation of 1.0 mmol/l, associate this K_M-value to the low sodium activated ouabain binding reported above. Therefore, the results might be explained by the assumption, that not only the phosphoenzyme facing outwards (E_2–P) but also the phosphoenzyme facing inwards (E_1–P) is capable of binding ouabain, if favourable ligand conditions are present. A similar differentiation of ouabain binding sites by sodium was also demonstrated in studies on the outer medulla of

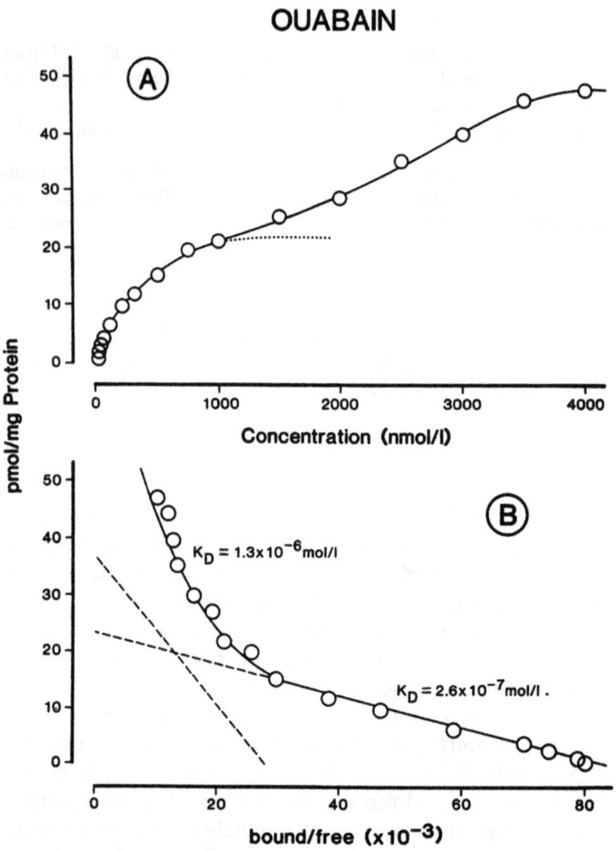

Fig. 1. Binding of ^{3}H-ouabain to guinea pig heart NaK-ATPase. Cardiac cell membranes (0.15 mg protein) incubated for 30 min at 37 °C in 100 mmol/l imidazole-HCl pH 7.4, 5 mmol/l $MgCl_2$, 3 mmol/l imidazole/PO_4^{3-}, 5.5 nmol/l ^{3}H-ouabain, and increasing concentrations of unlabelled ouabain (5×10^{-9} – 10^{-3} mol/l). Non-specific ^{3}H-ouabain binding in the presence of 10^{-3} mol/l unlabelled ouabain was subtracted. Further conditions as described under Methods and Materials.
A. Saturation binding of ^{3}H-ouabain. Mean of 6 different assays.
B. Scatchard plot of the same data, demonstrating two different populations of ouabain binding sites: A high affinity, low capacity binding site (B_{max} = 22.0 pmol/mg protein, $K_D = 2.6 \times 10^{-7}$ mol/l) and a low affinity, high capacity binding site (B_{max} = 37.0 pmol/mg protein, $K_D = 1.3 \times 10^{-6}$ mol/l), (Fricke, submitted).

canine kidney by Inagaki et al. (16). Furthermore, the results could also be extended to the more lipophilic steroids digoxin and digitoxin (11).

In order to get some more insight into the functional significance of the two ouabain binding sites operative in guinea pig heart NaK-ATPase, the results reported above were compared to both inhibition of this enzyme and cardiac glycoside induced inotropic action in guinea pig isolated papillary muscles (Table 1).

In cumulative dose-response curves, ouabain dose-dependently increased the contractile force in the range of 1×10^{-7} to 2×10^{-6} mol/l, with higher concentrations resulting in contracture and arrhythmias. Half maximal inotropic effects (ED_{50}) were obtained at 3.6 ×

Table 1. Ouabain induced increase in contractile force, inhibition of and binding to NaK-ATPase in guinea pig heart muscle

	Concentration ($\times 10^{-7}$mol/l)		n
ED_{50} (Inotropic action)	3.6		5
ID_{50} (Inhibition of NaK-ATPase)		10.9	6
K_D (Binding to NaK-ATPase)	2.6	13.2	6

Table 1. Concentrations of ouabain (mol/l) for half maximal increase in contractile force in guinea pig isolated papillary muscles (ED_{50}), half maximal inhibition of guinea pig heart NaK-ATPase (ID_{50}), and half maximal binding to guinea pig heart NaK-ATPase in the presence of Mg^{2+} and inorganic phosphate (K_D). Further conditions see Methods section or Figure 1, resp. Mean values out of "n" different experiments are shown (Fricke, unpublished).

10^{-7} mol/l (n = 5). NaK-ATPase activity of guinea pig heart, determined in separate experiments, was inhibited by ouabain concentrations beginning at 1×10^{-8}mol/l, with complete inhibition being obtained at 5×10^{-5} mol/l ouabain. The cardiac glycoside concentration for half maximal inhibition of the enzyme (ID_{50}) was calculated as 1.1×10^{-6} mol/l ouabain (n = 6).

Comparing these data with the dissociation constants obtained in the above mentioned binding studies (cf. fig 1), the high affinity, low capacity binding of ouabain to the NaK-ATPase seems to correlate with the inotropic action of this drug in guinea pig isolated papillary muscles, whereas the low affinity, high capacity binding of ouabain to the enzyme seems to be more related to the inhibition of the NaK-ATPase. These results are in agreement with the experiments and suggestions made by Erdmann and coworkers (5, 6) in rat and guinea pig heart (see above) that imply a dissociation of the cardiac glycoside induced inotropic action from the respective toxic events. This could be explained on the basis that the inotropic action of cardiac glycosides results from a conformational change of the NaK-ATPase leading finally to a "labilization" of membrane-bound calcium and/or subsequent changes of the cellular calcium binding characteristics (17, 19, 21), whereas the intoxication of the heart muscle is obtained at comparatively high ouabain concentrations only, which then result in an adequate NaK-ATPase-inhibition with subsequent impairment of the intra-, extracellular electrolyte balance.

Recently, the artificial food dye, erythrosin B, has been reported to selectively inhibit the high affinity ouabain binding to rat brain tissue (14, 23, 24). This hypothesis could be further tested by studying the erythrosin B/ouabain interaction in guinea pig heart muscle preparations. If – as outlined above – the high affinity, low capacity binding of ouabain to the NaK-ATPase is associated with the inotropic action of ouabain, this effect should be modified in the presence of erythrosin B, thereby discriminating the inotropic action of cardiac glycosides from their toxic manifestations.

In experiments on guinea pig heart Mg^{2+}-dependent, NaK-ATPase, erythrosin B proved to be a potent inhibitor of the ($Na^+ + K^+$)–, as well as Mg^{2+}-ATPase-activity with a concentration for half maximal inhibition of 9×10^{-6}mol/l (n = 3). The dissociation constant of erythrosin B was roughly in the same order ($K_D = 3.6 \times 10^{-6}$ mol/l, n = 6), as determined indirectly in the presence of Mg^{2+} and inorganic phosphate by inhibition of ^3H-ouabain binding to its binding site in guinea pig heart NaK-ATPase.

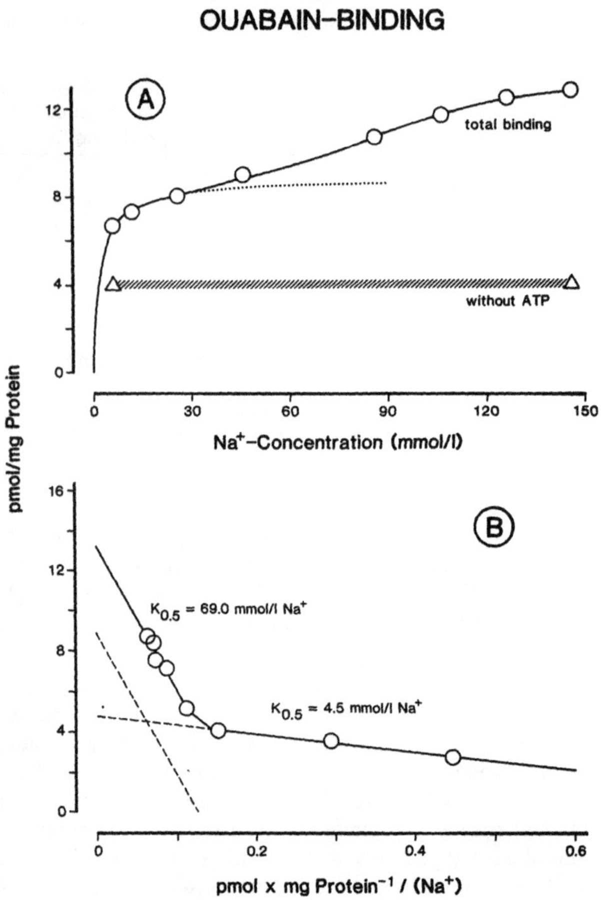

Fig. 2. Binding of ^{3}H-ouabain to guinea pig heart NaK-ATPase in the presence of increasing Na^+ concentrations. Cardiac cell membranes (0.3 mg protein) incubated for 30 min at 37 °C in 100 mmol/l imidazole-HCl pH 7.4, 5 mmol/l $MgCl_2$, various concentrations of NaCl (0–140 mmol/l), 1 mmol/l Na_2-EDTA, 5 nmol/l ^{3}H-ouabain, and 5×10^{-7} mol/l unlabelled ouabain in the presence (open circles) or absence (open triangles) of 2 mmol/l Na_2-ATP. Further conditions as described under Methods and Materials.

A. Na^+-dependence of ^{3}H-ouabain binding (5×10^{-7} mol/l).

Open circles represent total binding in the presence of ATP, open triangles ^{3}H-ouabain binding in the absence of ATP ("nonspecific binding"). Mean of 4 different assays.

B. Hofstee plot of the ATP-dependent ^{3}H-ouabain binding (nonspecific binding in the absence of ATP subtracted), demonstrating two different ouabain binding sites: A "high affinity Na^+-site", half maximal ouabain binding obtained at 4.5 mmol/l Na^+ (B_{max} = 4.7 pmol/mg protein), and a "low affinity Na^+-site" with half maximal ouabain binding demonstrable at 69 mmol/l Na^+ (B_{max} = 8.5 pmol/mg protein), data according to Fricke and Klaus (10).

If the ^{3}H-ouabain binding is now followed in the presence of different erythrosin B concentrations, which in the displacement studies depressed ouabain binding by about 60–80 %, a dose-dependent inhibition of the high affinity, low capacity ouabain binding can be demonstrated, whereas the low affinity, high capacity component remains uninfluenced (Table 2). So far, the results obtained in rat brain tissue (14, 23, 24) could also be confirmed in experiments on guinea pig heart NaK-ATPase.

Table 2. Inhibition of high affinity ouabain binding to guinea pig heart NaK-ATPase by erythrosin B

	Ouabain		
	–	+ Erythrosin B (5 × 10^{-6}mol/l)	+ Erythrosin B (1 × 10^{-5}mol/l)
High affinity sites			
B_{max} (pmol/mg protein)	11.9	11.8	–
K_D (× 10^{-7}mol/l)	2.0	4.3	–
Low affinity sites			
B_{max} (pmol/mg protein)	24.4	21.5	24.7
K_D (× 10^{-7}mol/l)	23.0	21.0	15.0

Table 2. Mg^{2+} and inorganic phosphate dependent ouabain binding to guinea pig heart NaK-ATPase in the presence or absence of different concentrations of erythrosin B (5 × 10^{-6} resp. 1 × 10^{-5} mol/l). Further conditions as in Figure 1. Data analyzed according to Scatchard (20). The means of 3–4 different experiments are given (Fricke, submitted).

However, when applied to the beating heart muscle preparation, erythrosin B in a concentration which completely inhibited the high affinity ouabain binding in the experiments mentioned above, did not alter ouabain induced inotropic action in isolated guinea pig atria (fig. 3).

Thus, from these experiments one might conclude that the high affinity, low capacity binding is *not* involved in ouabain induced positive inotropic action and – as the toxicity threshold under these conditions also remained uninfluenced – the low affinity, high capacity binding of the cardiac glycosides may be responsible for both the inotropic as well as the toxic action in guinea pig heart. With this reflection, however, the physiological significance of the high affinity binding of cardiac glycosides remains obscure. Therefore, the failure of erythrosin B to alter ouabain induced action in isolated guinea pig atria seems to be more related to a possible interference of erythrosin B with the ATP-site of the NaK-ATPase (24), which would suppose a cellular uptake of this drug, as yet not established.

Acknowledgements

The skillful technical assistance of Miss Sabine Bayer and Miss Iris Brebeck is gratefully appreciated.

References

1. Akera T, Brody TM (1977) The role of Na^+,K^+-ATPase in the inotropic action of digitalis. Pharmacol Rev 29:187–220
2. Brown L, Erdmann E, Thomas R (1983) Digitalis structure-activity relationship analyses. Conclusions from indirect binding studies with cardiac (Na^++K^+)-ATPase. Biochem Pharmacol 32:2767–2774

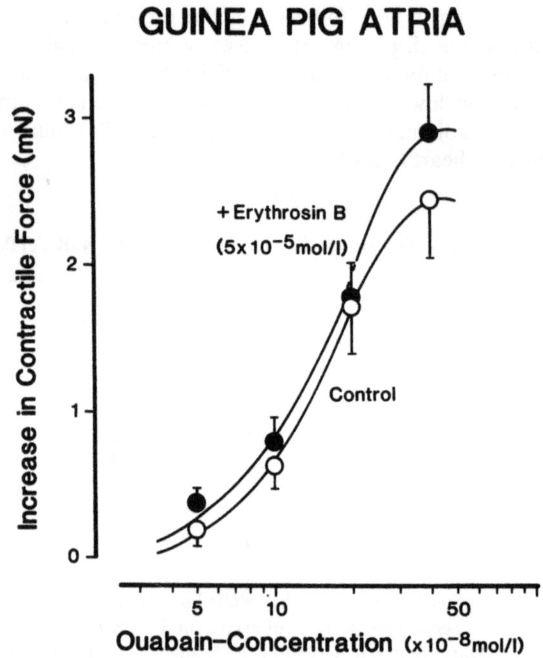

Fig. 3. Increase in contractile force (ordinate, in mN) in dependence on the ouabain concentration (abscissa, in mol/l) in the presence (closed circles) and absence (open circles) of 5×10^{-5} mol/l erythrosin B in isolated guinea pig left atria. Means ± S.E. means of 4 different experiments each are given (Fricke, submitted).

3. Eibl HJ, Lands WC (1969) A new sensitive determination of phosphate. Anal Biochem 30:51–57
4. Erdmann E (1981) Influence of cardiac glycosides on their receptor. In: Handbook of Experimental Pharmacology (Ed Greeff K), Springer Verlag, Berlin Heidelberg New York, Vol 56/I pp 337–380
5. Erdmann E (1983) Evidence for two kinetically and functionally different types of cardiac glycoside receptors in the heart. J Mol Cell Cardiol 15:(Suppl 2), 46
6. Erdmann E, Philipp G, Scholz H (1980) Cardiac glycoside receptor, $(Na^{+}+K^{+})$-ATPase activity and force of contraction in rat heart. Biochem Pharmacol 29:3219–3229
7. Erdmann E, Schoner W (1973) Ouabain-receptor interactions in $(Na^{+}+K^{+})$-ATPase preparations from different tissues and species. Determination of kinetic constants and dissociation constants. Biochim Biophys Acta 307:386–398
8. Erdmann, E, Schoner W (1974) Ouabain-receptor interactions in $(Na^{+}+K^{+})$-ATPase preparations. IV. The molecular structure of different cardioactive steroids and other substances and their affinity to the glycoside receptor. Naunyn-Schmiedebergs Arch Pharmacol 283:335–356
9. Fricke U, Klaus W (1974) A simple preparation technique for a microsomal Na^{+}–K^{+}-activated ATPase from cardiac tissues of different species. Prep Biochem 4:13–29
10. Fricke U, Klaus W (1977) Evidence for two different Na^{+}-dependent (^{3}H)-ouabain binding sites of a Na^{+}–K^{+}–ATPase of guinea-pig hearts. Brit J Pharmac 61:423–423
11. Fricke U, Klaus W (1978) Sodium-dependent cardiac glycoside binding: Experimental evidence and hypothesis. Brit J Parmac 62:255–257
12. Greeff K (1981) Handbook of Experimental Pharmacology, Vol 56/I Cardiac glycosides (Springer-Verlag, Berlin/Heidelberg/New York)
13. Hafner D, Heinen E, Noack E (1977) Mathematical analysis of concentration-response-relationships. Arneim-Forsch 27:1871–1873

14. Hnatowich M, LaBella FS (1982) Light-enhanced inhibition of ouabain binding to digitalis receptor in rat brain and guinea pig heart by the food dye erythrosine. Mol Pharmacol 22:687–692
15. Hofstee BHJ (1952) On the evaluation of the constants V_m and K_m in enzyme reactions. Science 116:329–331
16. Inagaki C, Lindenmayer GE, Schwartz A (1974) Effects of sodium and potassium on binding of ouabain to the transport adenosine triphosphatase. J Biol Chem 249:513–5140
17. Klaus W, Fricke U (1978) Electrolyte-dependence of cardiac glycoside actions at the cellular and subcellular level. In: Kobayashi T, Sano T, Dhalla NS (eds) Recent advances in studies on cardiac structure and metabolism, Vol 11, Heart function and metabolism. University Park Press, Baltimore pp 393–399
18. Lowry OH, Rosebrough NJ, Farr AF, Randall RJ (1951) Protein measurement with the folin phenol reagent. J Biol Chem 193:265–275
19. Lüllmann H, Peters T (1979) Action of cardiac glycosides on the excitation-contraction coupling in heart muscle. Progr Pharmacol 2:1–53
20. Scatchard G (1949) The attractions of proteins for small molecules and ions. NY Acad Sci (USA) 51:660–672
21. Schwartz A (1976) Is the cell membrane Na^+,K^+-ATPase enzyme system the pharmacological receptor for digitalis? Circul Res 39:2–7
22. Schwartz A, Lindenmayer GE, Allen JC (1975) The sodium-potassium adenosine triphosphatase: Pharmacological, physiological and biochemical aspects. Pharmacol Rev 27:3–134
23. Silbergeld EK (1981) Erythrosin B is a specific inhibitor of high affinity ^{3}H-ouabain binding and ion transport in rat brain. Neuropharmacol 20:87–90
24. Swann AC (1982) Brain (Na^+–K^+)-ATPase: Biphasic interaction with erythrosin B. Biochem Pharmacol 31:2185–2190

Author's address:

Uwe Fricke, Pharmakologisches Institut der Universität zu Köln, Gleueler Str. 24, D-5000 Köln 41 (FRG)

Effects of calcium on the heterogeneity of the Na^+, K^+-ATPase forms in rat heart

L. G. Lelievre, P. Mansier, D. Charlemagne, and B. Swynghedauw

INSERM U 127, Université Paris 7, Hôpital Lariboisière, Paris (France)

Summary

The sensitivity of the Na^+, K^+-ATPase to ouabain has been studied in sarcolemma vesicles isolated from normal rat heart. Two enzyme forms exhibiting high and low sensitivities to ouabain have been observed in Ca^{2+}-free perfused heart. The half-maximal inhibitory effects occurred with $1–2 \times 10^{-8}$M ouabain. The high sensitivity form undetectable in hearts maintained at a physiological Ca^{2+} level might represent altered low affinity sites or latent enzyme forms unmasked by low calcium concentrations.

The heterogeneity of the Na^+, K^+-ATPase forms was found to be also modulated by the K^+/ouabain antagonism, addition of K^+ accentuating the heterogeneity.

These *in vitro* results associated with *in vivo* experiments on isolated rat heart working under isovolumic conditions suggested that lowering Ca^{2+} has qualitative and quantitative effects. Low Ca^{2+} concentrations increased the sensitivities to ouabain and the amplitudes of both the enzyme inhibition and the positive inotropic effects.

Key words: rat cardiac sarcolemma-Ca^{2+}-sensitivity Na^+, K^+-ATPase-ouabain, $(Na^+ + K^+)$-ATPase, cardiac glycosides, rat heart, calcium

Introduction

In the last decade, a large body of evidence, mainly based upon kinetic studies, introduced and strengthened the concept that membrane-bound receptors were or would be heterogeneous, at least, in their affinities for one of their specific ligands. Thus, in tissues and species such as rat brain (6, 21), rat heart (1, 4, 5, 15, 17), dog heart (23) or guinea-pig heart (10) and ligands as different as endogenous opiates (6) or exogenous digitalis (1, 4, 5, 10, 15, 17, 23), the specific receptors were found to be heterogeneous. The physiological relevance of this dual expression remains questionable.

The ouabain-receptors at the cardiac cell surface have been characterized by comparison of the dose-response curves of the positive inotropic effect *in vivo* with those of both the ^{3}H-ouabain-binding and the Na^+, K^+-ATPase (or Na^+-pump) inhibition *in vitro*. It is generally admitted that the pharmacologically active digitalis concentrations correlate with the sensitivities of the cardiac Na^+, K^+-ATPases to inhibition by ouabain.

Until a few years ago, it was thought that the rat cardiac enzyme consisted of an homogeneous population insensitive to ouabain with K_D's for binding and half-maximal inhibition in the range of $1–6 \times 10^{-5}$M (1, 4, 20, 21). However recently, Erdmann et al. (4) reported that two ^{3}H ouabain-binding sites did exist in rat heart: high affinity sites (K_D = $1–2.3 \times 10^{-7}$M) associated with the increase in force of contraction and low affinity sites (K_D = 2.8×10^{-5}M) related to both Na^+-pump inhibition and cardiac arrythmias.

These results were partially confirmed by Adams et al. (1) who found two classes of ^{3}H-ouabain-binding sites both related to positive inotropic effects in vivo. Again, the Na^+,

K^+-ATPase inhibition was found to be associated with the occupancy of low affinity sites. Thus, according to these authors, the rat cardiac sarcolemma specifically binds ouabain with no detectable concomitant enzyme inhibition. This conclusion is controversial since we recently showed that high affinity ouabain-binding sites were associated with a Na^+, K^+-ATPase activity provided the calcium concentration was decreased (15, 17).

The present paper is concerned with the role(s) played by Ca^{2+} and K^+ ions in the expression of the heterogeneity of the Na^+, K^+-ATPase activities assayed in fractions highly enriched in sarcolemmal vesicles. In parallel, we analyzed the consequences of low Ca^{2+} perfusions on the force of contraction induced by ouabain in working rat heart.

The results clearly showed that lowering Ca^{2+} *in vivo* or increasing K^+ *in vitro* accentuated the heterogeneity of the ouabain-receptors.

Methods

1. Isolation of a highly enriched sarcolemmal fraction

Hearts isolated from male Wistar rats (240–300 g) were depleted of calcium or maintained at a normal calcium concentration (2mM). In the former case, the heart was completely relaxed by perfusion of either an EDTA-containing relaxing buffer (15, 16) (pCa 8) or with a Ca^{2+}-free Krebs-Ringer bicarbonate buffer (pCa 4.7) (19). To maintain a physiological Ca^{2+} concentration, the perfusion was either omitted or performed with a Ca^{2+}-containing buffer. Sarcolemmal vesicles were isolated by differential centrifugations according to Mansier et al. (16) or Jorgensen and Skou (11).

The ventricles were homogenized at 4 °C in 30 ml of 20 mM sodium pyrophosphate (PP_i), 0.1 mM phenylmethane sulfonylfluoride, 10 mM Tris-HCl pH 7.8 with a Polytron PT 20 (2 × 0.5 sec. setting 5). After a 20 min. period stirring at 4° C, the suspension was made up 120 mM KCl, 30 mM NaCl and 250 mM sucrose by adding concentrated solutions. The 500 × g – 5 min. supernatant was diluted to 120 ml of this isotonic and isoosmotic solution adjusted to pH 6.8 with 40 mM Imidazole – HCl (Buffer I) and centrifuged successively at 7,500 × g for 15 min. and at 31,000 × g for 30 min. The final pellet (P_2) was washed in 50 mM PP_i, 135 mM NaCl, 5 mM $MgCl_2$ and 5 mM Tris-HCl pH 7.4 to eliminate myofibrils. The washed microsomes resuspended in Buffer I were layered over 30 % sucrose solution and centrifuged for 90 min. at 100,000 × g (16). The top layer (G_2) was recovered, diluted with 3 volumes of 100 mM NaCl and 40 mM Imidazole-HCl pH 6.8 and centrifuged at 31,000 × g for 30 min. The pellet (P_2) was resuspended in this buffer supplemented with 250 mM sucrose.

The method of Jorgensen and Skou (11) applied to rat heart differed from that of Mansier et al. (16) in that i) the homogenization with a Polytron was carried out under isoosmotic conditions (250 mM sucrose and 30 mM Imidazole – HCl pH 6.8) and ii) the 20 min-period stirring at 4 °C was omitted.

2. Estimation of Na^+,K^+-ATPase activity

The Na^+, K^+-ATPase activity was assayed as previously described (15, 16) using 10 µg protein/ml incubation medium (14). The sarcolemmal vesicles were preincubated with ouabain (Boehringer) for 30 min at 37 °C with or without 10 mM KCl in the assay medium containing 4 mM $MgCl_2$, 100 mM NaCl and 40 mM Imidazole-HCl (pH 7.4). The reaction was then initiated with the addition of either ATP or ATP + KCl (final concentrations: 4 or 4 and 10 mM, respectively) and carried out over 6 time points to assess linearity. Every 30 sec, aliquots were taken and the released orthophosphate was measured (3).

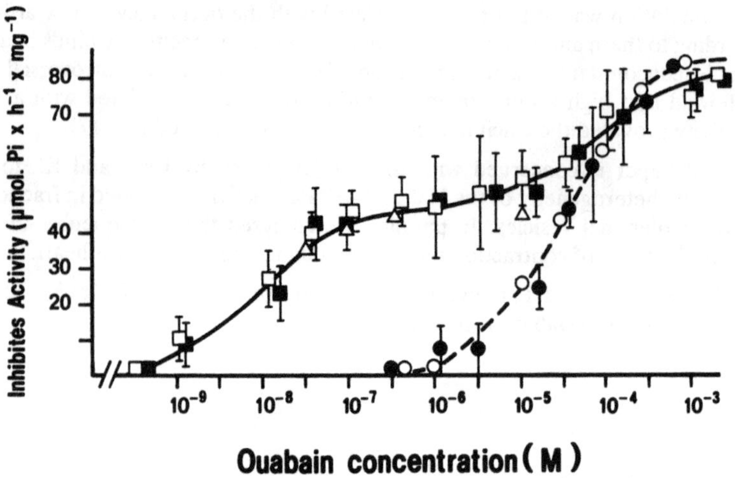

Fig. 1 Dose-response curves of Na^+, K^+-ATPase activity versus ouabain concentration. Dotted curve : heart maintained at 2 mM Ca^{2+} : native (●) and opened (○) sarcolemmal vesicles. Solid curve : Ca^{2+}-free perfused heart : native (■) and opened (□) sarcolemmal vesicles, opened vesicles subfractionated on sucrose (Δ).

In the microsomes, the Na^+, K^+-ATPase activities represented 50 ± 10% of the total ATPase activities. This proportion increased to 75 ± 5% in highly enriched sarcolemmal vesicles (G_2). The Na^+, K^+-ATPase was measured before and after unmasking the total activity with sodium dodecyl sulfate (16) or by reiterative freezings and thawings (15, 16). These assays in the presence of ATP, which favours ouabain binding, were linear with respect to time, suggesting that the enzyme-ouabain equilibrium was reached in less than 1 min (the shortest time used).

Results

The preparations used here were highly enriched in sarcolemmal vesicles. The specific activities of Na^+, K^+-ATPase averaged 85 ± 15 or 100 ± 20 µmol.Pi × h^{-1} × mg^{-1} whatever the isolation procedure or the heart pretreatment. Note that the yields in microsomal (or sarcolemmal) proteins were up to 50% lower than those from hearts perfused with Ca^{2+}-free buffers whereas the specific activity of the Na^+, K^+-ATPase remained constant.

Native and opened sarcolemmal vesicles from Ca^{2+}-free perfused hearts exhibited a two-step dose-response curve to ouabain (Fig. 1 and 2): 45 to 65% of the enzyme activity was inhibited between 10^{-9} and 3×10^{-7}M ouabain, the half-maximal inhibition (IC_{50}) occurring between 1 and 2×10^{-8}M ouabain. A plateau associated with 35–55% of the total activity was found between 3×10^{-7} and 10^{-5}M. Fifty per cent inhibition of this residual activity was obtained with doses varying from 3 to 8×10^{-5}M ouabain. A similar biphasic curve was obtained with sarcolemma vesicles further purified by centrifugation on sucrose. (Specific activity of Na^+, K^+-ATPase: 200 ± 20 µmol. phosphate h^{-1}. mg^{-1}).

Opened and native sarcolemmal vesicles from hearts maintained at a physiological Ca^{2+} yielded a homogeneous population of Na^+, K^+-ATPase exhibiting a low sensitivity to ouabain (IC_{50}: 4 ± 2 × 10^{-5}M) (dotted curves in Fig. 1 and 2).

In order to study the reactivity of these enzyme forms to K^+/ouabain antagonism, the same experiments have been carried out under conditions in which K^+ was omitted during the preincubation with ouabain. Potassium was added simultaneously with ATP to initiate the enzymatic reaction. As shown in Fig. 2 the K^+/ouabain antagonism was much more pronounced in Ca^{2+}-free perfused hearts than in hearts maintained at the physiological Ca^{2+} level. The absence of K^+ resulted in a partial conversion of the low sensitivity form into the high sensitivity one. The activity associated with the low sensitivity enzyme form represented about 15 % of the total Na^+, K^+-ATPase activity.

Discussion

The results presented here clearly demonstrated that a Ca^{2+}-free perfusion of rat heart revealed a heterogeneous population of active Na^+, K^+-ATPase forms. The analysis of this heterogeneity depends upon the criteria chosen to express the enzyme activity, i.e.: the specific activity or the total activity (specific activity x protein yield).

As the specific activity of the Na^+, K^+-ATPase was constant, whatever the heart pretreatment, one might suppose that the high sensitivity form represented low sensitivity forms altered by the Ca^{2+}-free perfusion and/or the procedure of isolation may have changed the properties of the enzyme in relation to the effect of glycoside, that is an increased sensitivity (12, 13, 22, 24). If the enzyme activity was expressed in terms of total activity (Fig. 3), the Na^+, K^+-ATPase in Ca^{2+}-free perfused heart preparations largely exceeded that found in Ca^{2+}-containing hearts. The increment of activity was mainly, if not exclusively, associated with the high sensitivity form. Our interpretations would be that in hearts maintained at a physiological Ca^{2+} level, the high sensitivity form was either lost or existed as a catalytically inactive conformation as suggested by Adams et al. (1)

The biological relevance in terms of inotropy (7, 8, 18) of these high and low sensitivity Na^+,K^+-ATPase forms as a function of the Ca^{2+} concentrations has been studied on isolated rat heart working under isovolumic conditions. This model is quite different from that used by Erdmann et al. (4) and Adams et al. (1) i.e. isometric contraction of ventricular strips. In agreement with the earlier observations of Fricke et al. (8), preliminary experiments carried out in our laboratory showed that:

i) ouabain, even at high concentrations (up to 10^{-4}M) did not activate contractility when the total concentration of Ca^{2+} of the perfusate was above 0.5 mM;

ii) at this low Ca^{2+} level, ouabain (as low as 10^{-8}M) significantly increased the speed of shortening (dP/dt) and the dP/dt $\times$ P^{-1} (as an index of inotropy) and

iii) the amplitudes of the observed effects were increased reaching about 400 % above control instead of 80 to 100 % according to several authors (1, 2, 4, 5, 7, 18, 23).

Thus, low Ca^{2+} concentrations have both qualitative and quantitative effects. Lowering Ca^{2+} revealed a sarcolemma-bound Na^+, K^+-ATPase activity highly sensitive to ouabain and greatly increased the sensitivity of the whole rat heart to the drug. Quantitatively, at a given ouabain concentration, a decrease in Ca^{2+} resulted in an enhancement of both the degree of enzyme inhibition *in vitro* and the amplitude of the positive inotropic effect *in vivo*.

Whether these effects of Ca^{2+} are due to the existence of isoenzymic forms of Na^+, K^+-ATPase (21) differently affected by Ca^{2+} (8, 15, 17) or to a role of Ca^{2+}-binding elements linked to the sarcolemma (9, 12, 13, 24) remains an open question.

Acknowledgements

The authors are very grateful to Mrs. M. Preteseille and Mr. C. Mouas for technical assistance.

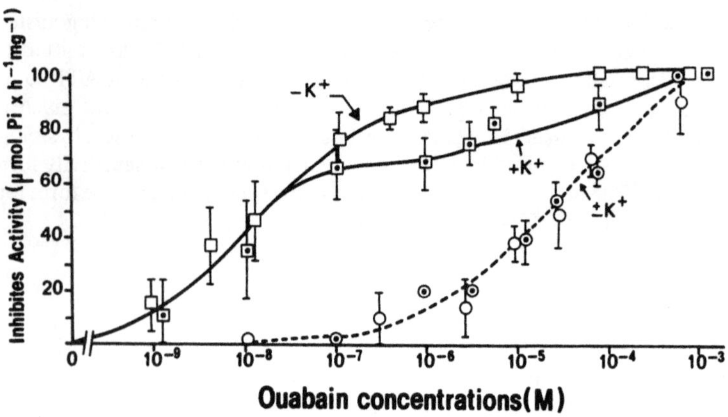

Fig. 2 Dose-response curves of Na^+, K^+-ATPase activity versus ouabain concentration in microsomes. Dotted curves : hearts maintained at 2 mM Ca^{2+}, microsomes preincubated without K^+ (○) or with 10 mK K^+ (⊙). Solid curves : Ca^{2+}-free perfused hearts, microsomes preincubated without K^+ (□) or with 10 mM K^+ (⊡).

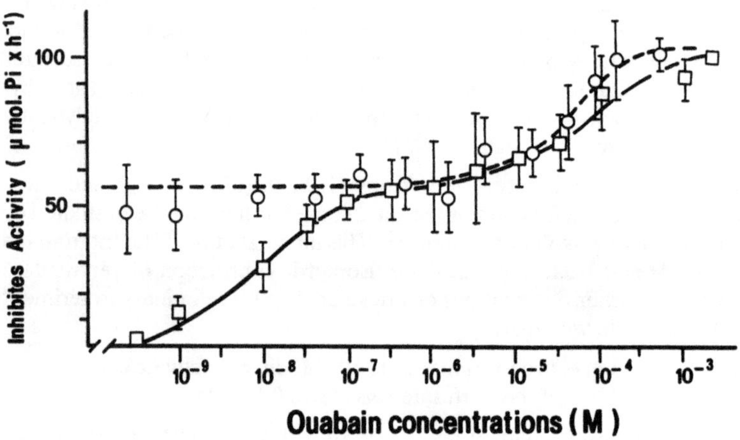

Fig. 3 Dose-response curve of *total* Na^+, K^+-ATPase activities versus ouabain concentration in microsomes from heart maintained at 2 mM Ca^{2+} (○) or from Ca^{2+}-free perfused heart (□). Total activity : specific activity × protein yield. The protein yield was arbitrarily set at 1 in Ca^{2+}-free perfused hearts. For a better visualization of a possible unmasking effect of low (Ca^{2+}) on the high sensitivity enzyme form, the origin of the dotted curve has been shifted to the top on the ordinate axis by 50 ± 14 units.

References

1. Adams RJ, Schwartz A, Grupp G, Grupp I, Lee SW, Wallick ET, Powell T, Twist VW, Gathiram P (1982) High-affinity binding site and low-dose positive inotropic effect in rat myocardium. Nature 296:167–169
2. Akera T, Brody TM (1982) Myocardial Membranes: Regulation and function of the sodium pump. Ann Rev Physiol 44:375–388

3. Anner B, Moosmayer M (1975) Rapid determination of inorganic phosphate in biological systems by a highly sensitive photometric method. Anal Biochem 65:305–309
4. Erdmann E, Philipp G, Scholz H (1980) Cardiac glycoside receptor, $(Na^+ + K^+)$-ATPase activity and force of contraction in rat heart. Biochem Pharmacol 29:3219–3229
5. Finet M, Noel F, Godfraind T (1982) Inotropic effect and binding sites of ouabain to rat heart. Arch Intern Pharmacodyn Ther 256:168–170
6. Fischel SV, Medzihradsky F (1981) Scatchard analysis of opiate receptor binding. Mol Pharmacol 20:269–279
7. Fricke U, Klaus W (1977) Evidence for two different Na^+-dependent ^3H-ouabain binding sites of a (Na^+,K^+)-ATPase of guinea-pig hearts. Br J Pharmacol 61:423–428
8. Fricke U, Klaus W, Majunke HJ (1982) Effects of calcium on ouabain-induced inotropism in rat and guinea-pig hearts. In: Advances in Myocardiology. Vol 3 pp 27–31. Ed Chavoz E, Smirnov V and Dhalla NS. Plenum Publishing Corporation
9. Geny B, Paraf A, Fedon Y, Charlemagne D (1982) Characterization of a B actinin-like protein in purified non-muscle cell membranes. Biochim Biophys Acta 692:345–354
10. Godfraind T, de Pover A, Tona Lutete DN (1980) Identification with potassium and vanadate of two classes of specific ouabain binding sites in a $(Na^+ + K^+)$-ATPase preparation from the guinea-pig heart. Biochem Pharmacol 29:1195–1199
11. Jorgensen PL, Skou JC (1969) Preparation of highly active $(Na^+ + K^+)$-ATPase from the outer medulla of rabbit kidney. Biochem Biophys Res Commun 37:39–46
12. Lelievre LG, Zachowski A, Charlemagne D, Laget P, Paraf A (1979) Involvement of membrane proteins and Ca^{2+} in the sensitivity of $(Na^+ + K^+)$-ATPase to ouabain. Biochim Biophys Acta 557:399–408
13. Lelievre LG, Piascik MT, Potter JD, Wallick ET, Schwartz A (1983) Involvement of Calmodulin in the inhibition of Na, K-ATPase by ouabain. In: Current Topics in Membranes and Transport. Vol 19 pp 1023–1027. Ed Forbush B. and Hoffman J. F. Academic Press. New York.
14. Lowry OH, Rosebrough NJ, Farr AL, Randall RJ (1951) Protein measurement with the Folin phenol reagent. J Biol Chem 193:265–275
15. Mansier P, Lelievre LG (1982) Ca^{2+}-free perfusion of rat heart reveals a $(Na^+ + K^+)$-ATPase form highly sensitive to ouabain. Nature, 300, 535–537
16. Mansier P, Charlemagne D, Rossi B, Preteseille M, Swynghedauw, Lelievre LG (1983) Isolation of impermeable inside-out vesicles from an enriched sarcolemma fraction of rat heart. J Biol Chem 258:6628–6635
17. Mansier P, Cassidy PS, Charlemagne D, Preteseille M, Lelievre LG (1983) Three Na^+, K^+-ATPase forms in rat heart as revealed by K^+/ouabain antagonism. FEBS Letters 153:357–360 (1983)
18. Noble D (1980) Mechanism of action of therapeutic levels of cardiac glycosides. Cardiovasc Res 14: 495–514
19. Powell T, Terrar DA, Twist VW (1980) Electrical properties of individual cells isolated from adult rat ventricular myocardium. J Physiol 302:131–153
20. Repke K (1965) Effects of digitalis on membrane adenosine triphosphatase of cardiac muscle. In: Proc of the IInd International Pharmacological Meeting. Drugs and Enzymes Vol 4 pp 65–87. Ed Brodie BB and Gillette JR
21. Sweadner K (1979) Two molecular forms of Na^+, K^+-ATPase in brain; Separation and difference in affinity for strophanthidin. J Biol Chem 254:6060–6067
22. Schwalb H, Dickstein Y, Heller M (1982) Interactions of cardiac glycosides with cardiac cells. III. Alterations in the sensitivity of Na^+, K^+ ATPase to inhibition by ouabain in rat hearts. Biochim Biophys Acta 689:241–248
23. Wellsmith NV, Lindenmayer GE (1980) Two receptor forms for ouabain in sarcolemma-enriched preparations from canine ventricles. Circ Res 47:710–720
24. Zachowski A, Lelievre LG, Aubry J, Charlemagne D, Paraf A (1977) Roles of proteins from inner face of plasma membranes in susceptibility of Na^+, K^+-ATPase to ouabain. Proc Natl Acad Sci USA 74:633–637

Authors' address:

Dr. L. G. Lelievre, INSERM U 127 – Université Paris 7, Hôpital Lariboisière, 41 Boulevard de la Chapelle, F-7 50 10 Paris

Positive inotropic effects of digitoxin- and digoxin-glucuronide in human isolated ventricular heart muscle preparations

H. Scholz and W. Schmitz

Abteilung Allgemeine Pharmakologie, Universitäts-Krankenhaus Eppendorf, Hamburg (FRG)

Summary

The effect on force of contraction of human isolated ventricular heart muscle preparations was studied with the 16′-glucuronides of digitoxin (dt-gluc) and digoxin (dg-gluc). The parent compounds digitoxin (dt) and digoxin (dg) were studied for comparison and all compounds were also investigated in guinea-pig isolated papillary muscles. All compounds increased myocardial force of contraction in human preparations in a concentration-dependent manner. The positive inotropic effect of dt-gluc and dg-gluc began at 0.1 $\mu mol\ l^{-1}$ and was maximal at 1 $\mu mol\ l^{-1}$. The metabolites were slightly less potent but, on the other hand, slightly more effective than the parent compounds dt and dg. The positive inotropic effects of all compounds peaked after about 60 minutes. In contrast, the decline of the positive inotropic effect upon washing was about twice as fast in the case of the hydrophilic metabolites. Similar results were obtained in guinea-pig papillary muscles. It is concluded that the glucuronides of digitoxin and digoxin are biologically active in the human heart. This may be of clinical importance with respect to the positive inotropic action and the plasma level determination of the cardiac glycosides.

Key words: digitoxin-glucuronide, digoxin-glucuronide, positive inotropic effect, human heart

Introduction

The metabolism of cardiac glycosides comprises the following steps (Rietbrock and Woodcock 1981, Storstein 1981):

1. Cleavage of the digitoxose residues,
2. conjugation reactions,
3. hydroxylation and
4. reduction of unsaturated lactone rings.

Among these enzymatic pathways, conjugation with glucuronic acid has been shown to be significant in the elimination of cardiac glycosides in man, at least in the case of digitoxin, both on maintenance treatment and after a single dose (Storstein 1981). However, it is still a matter of debate whether such conjugation products are still cardioactive. In guinea-pig atria, conjugated metabolic products of digitoxin and digoxin did not produce any alteration in force of contraction (Lüllmann and Peters 1971). In contrast, glucuronides of several digitalis glycosides have been shown to have inotropic properties in guinea-pig papillary muscles (Belz and Heinz 1977), but conjugated metabolites are generally believed to be inactive in man. The present study was designated to investigate whether conjugated metabolites of cardiac glycosides are capable of increasing the force of contraction of ventricular heart muscle preparations isolated from man. The inotropic effects of the hydrophilic metabolites of the tridigitoxosides digitoxin and digoxin were studied with digitoxin-16′-glucuronide and digoxin-16′-glucuronide as examples which have been synthetized for research purposes (Petersen et al. 1977). For comparison the effects of these compounds were also studied in guinea-pig papillary muscles.

Methods

Human heart muscle preparations were obtained from patients during open heart surgery*. Adult patients ranged in age from 21–60 years (mean 49.5 years) and children were 2–24 months old (mean 11.5 months). Heart diseases in the adult group consisted of atrial septal defect, mitral valve stenosis and Fallot's tetralogy whereas the children suffered from various congenital lesions. The patients were on treatment with beta-acetyldigoxin and diuretics, but drug therapy had been withdrawn one day before operation. General anaesthesia was performed with etomidate, fentanyl, droperidol and pancuronium. Cardiac surgery was generally performed on cardiopulmonary bypass and cardioplegic arrest. The cardioplegic solution had the following composition (mmol l^{-1}): NaCl 147.0, $CaCl_2$ 2.16, $MgCl_2$ 16.0, KCl 19.9, procaine HCl 1.0. The heart muscle preparations which were obtained from the right ventricle or the ventricular septum were placed in cold (4 °C) aerated bathing solution (composition see below) immediately after excision and delivered to the laboratory. The time between excision and the beginning of the laboratory processing was about 30 min. In order to minimize inadequate oxygenation the preparations were split into thin strips of not more than 1 mm thickness. This dissection was performed in aerated bathing solution at room temperature and was carried out so that the fibres in the preparations ran parallel to the length of the strips. The thickness of the muscle strips ranged from 0.6 to 1.0 mm and their length from 4.2 to 7.0 mm. Each strip was attached to a bipolar platinum stimulating electrode and suspended individually in glass tissue chambers for recording isometric contractions (for details see Meinertz et al. 1976). The bathing solution (75 ml) containing (mmol l^{-1}) NaCl 136.9, KCl 5.4, $CaCl_2$ 1.8, $MgCl_2$ 1.05, NaH_2PO_4 0.42, $NaHCO_3$ 11.9, Na_2EDTA 0.05, ascorbic acid 0.28, glucose 5.5 was continuously gassed with 95% O_2 + 5% CO_2 and maintained at 35 °C; the pH was 7.4. The force of contraction was measured with an inductive force transducer (W. Fleck, Mainz) attached to a Hellige Helco skriptor recorder. Resting force was adjusted to and maintained at 4 mN. The preparations were electrically paced at 0.5 Hz with rectangular pulses of 5 ms duration (Grass stimulator SD9); the voltage was about 20% greater than threshold. All preparations were allowed to equilibrate for at least 2 hours before any drug addition. All drugs were freshly dissolved in pre-warmed and pre-aerated bathing solution. Concentration-response curves were obtained cumulatively. The time of exposure to each drug concentration was 60 min. Force of contraction was measured immediately before any drug addition (predrug value) and after 60 min of exposure to each drug concentration.

Guinea-pig papillary muscles were obtained from the right ventricles. The animals (either sex; body weight 280–480 g) were killed by a blow on the head and bled from the carotid arteries. Their hearts were quickly excised and the papillary muscles (diameter 0.7–1.0 mm; length 3.0–6.0 mm) were dissected in aerated bathing solution at room temperature. The further experimental procedure was the same as described above for the human heart muscle strips except that the time of exposure to each drug concentration was 30 min.

Drugs used were digitoxin and digoxin from Merck (Darmstadt). Digitoxin-16'-glucuronide (dt-gluc, Na salt) and digoxin-16'-glucuronide (dg-gluc, Na salt) were kindly supplied by Dr. H. Flasch, Department of Clinical Research, Beiersdorf AG, Hamburg. Digitoxin and digoxin were dissolved in 70% ethanol and diluted with bathing solution. The final ethanol concentration in the organ bath was less than 0.1% and without any effect. The metabolites were directly dissolved in bathing solution.

All experimental values are given as means ± S.E.M. Statistical comparisons were performed with Student's t-test. A p-value of less than 0.05 was considered significant.

Results

The hydrophilic metabolites dt-gluc and dg-gluc produced a concentration-dependent positive inotropic effect. The results, together with those obtained with the parent compounds dt and dg, are summarized in Fig. 1. The positive inotropic effect of dt-gluc (Fig. 1A) began at a concentration of 0.1 μmol l^{-1} and was maximal at 1 μmol l^{-1}. The half-maximally effective concentration (EC_{50}) amounted to 0.37 μmol l^{-1}. The maximal increase in force of contraction

* The surgical specimens of the heart were generously supplied by Prof. Dr. H. Oelert, Division of Cardiac Surgery, Medizinische Hochschule Hannover.

was 378 ± 98% (n = 4) of the predrug values. Higher concentrations produced contractures and aftercontractions as a sign of toxicity within 15 min in all cases (marked by asterisks in Fig. 1). As compared to the parent compound dt, dt-gluc appeared to be slightly more effective and slightly less potent, but these differences did not reach the level of significance. Fig. 1B shows that effects similar to those of dt-gluc and dt were obtained with dg-gluc and dg. The difference in the maximal effects of dg-gluc and dg was somewhat less pronounced than in the case of dt-gluc and dt, but the difference in potency between the metabolite and the parent compound was significant (EC_{50} 0.46 vs. 0.26 μmol l^{-1}, $p < 0.05$).

The time course of the positive inotropic effect of these agents was studied with the EC_{75} of each compound, i.e. with concentrations which produced 75% of the maximal effect. These concentrations were chosen in order to obtain well-pronounced positive inotropic but no toxic effects. It is evident from the typical examples shown in Fig. 2 that the positive inotropic effects of all drugs developed gradually and reached their peaks after about 60 min. It is also evident that there were virtually no differences in the rate with which the effects of the parent compounds and the metabolites developed. In contrast, however, the decline of the positive inotropic effect upon washing in drug-free solution was about twice as fast in the case of the hydrophilic metabolites. For a complete return to the predrug values, dt-gluc and dg-gluc likewise required a washing period of about 6 hours whereas about 11 hours were needed for dt and dg in these preparations.

Roughly similar results were obtained in electrically driven guinea-pig papillary muscles (Fig. 3). Again, the metabolites tended to be more effective than the parent compounds. In

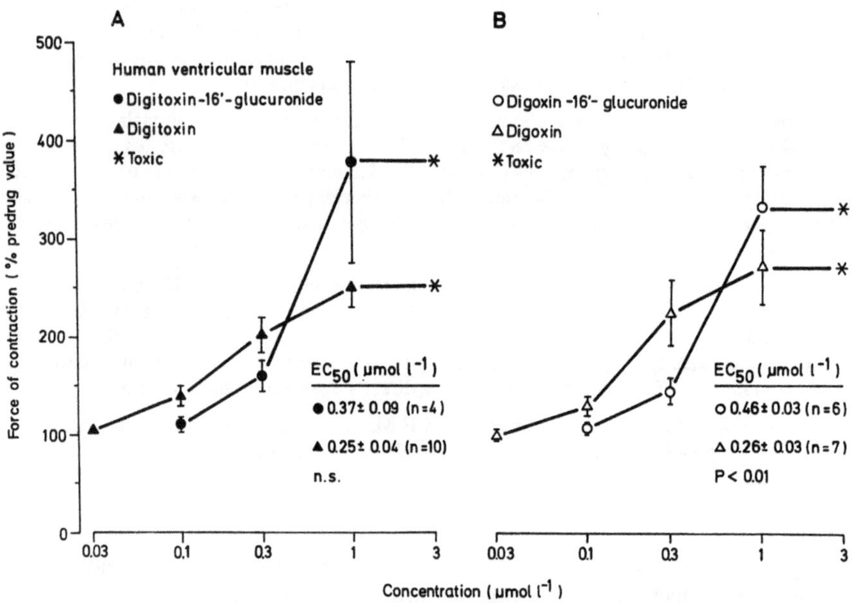

Fig. 1. Effect of dt-gluc (●), dt (▲), dg-gluc (○) and dg (△) on force of contraction of human isolated ventricular heart muscle strips. The concentration-response curves were obtained cumulatively with an incubation period of 60 minutes for each concentration. Toxic concentrations of the compounds (contractures and aftercontractions within 15 minutes in all cases) are visualized by asterisks. EC_{50} = concentration which produced 50 per cent of the maximal effect. The predrug values were 1.96 ± 0.25 mN (n = 27)

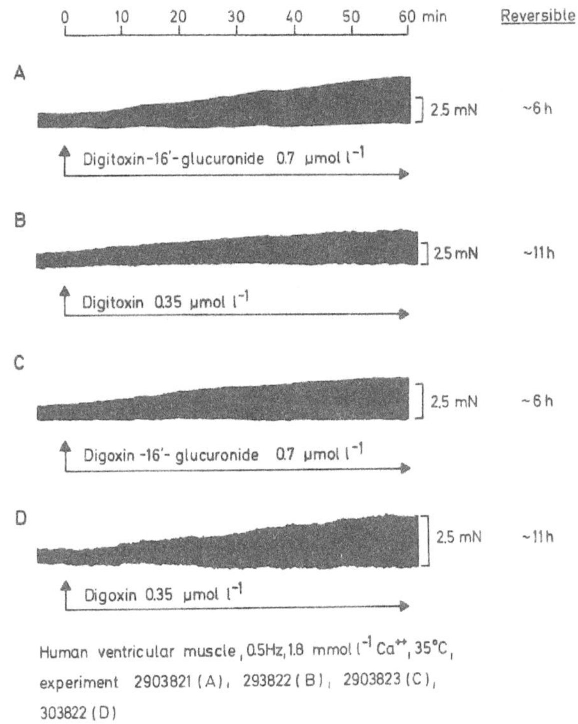

Fig. 2. Original tracings illustrating force of contraction of human isolated ventricular heart muscle strips before and 60 minutes after addition of dt-gluc (A), dt (B), dg-gluc (C) and dg (D). The concentrations investigated correspond to the EC_{75} values of each compound (concentrations to produce 75% of the maximal effect) as obtained from the concentration-response curves of Fig. 1. After washing with drug-free buffer, the positive inotropic response was completely reversible after about 6 hours in A and C (metabolites) and after about 11 hours in B and D (parent compounds).

the case of dt-gluc, this difference was significant (maximal increase in force of contraction to 953% and to 457% of control respectively; $p < 0.01$). On the other hand, dg-gluc was about 4 times less potent than dg (EC_{50} 4.43 and 1.08 µmol l^{-1}) whereas the potency of dt-gluc and dt were the same. The time course of the effects was again studied with the EC_{75} of each compound (1.5 µmol l^{-1} dt-gluc, dt and dg; 7 µmol l^{-1} dg-gluc). It was found that the build-up of the positive inotropic effects of the metabolites was somewhat slower than in the case of dt and dg; maximal responses were reached after about 50 min (metabolites) and 30 min (parent compounds) respectively. In contrast, the positive inotropic effects of the hydrophilic metabolites declined faster upon washing. The effects of dt-gluc and dg-gluc were completely reversible after about 1 hour whereas at least 2 hours were required in the case of dt and dg. Thus, the reversibility of all effects was appreciably faster in guinea-pig than in human preparations, but in both species the effects of the metabolites similarly declined faster by a factor of about 2 (6 vs. 11 hours in human and 1 vs. 2 hours in guinea-pig preparations).

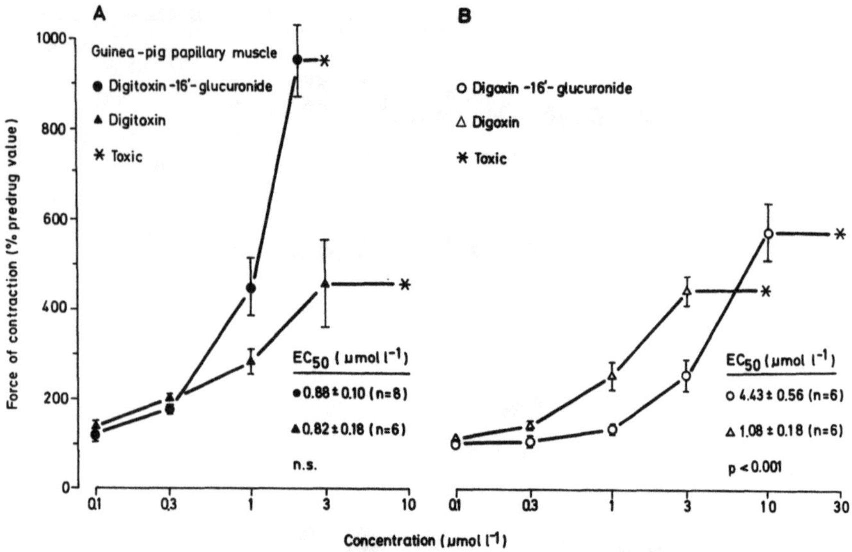

Fig. 3. Effect of dt-gluc (●), dt (▲), dg-gluc (○) and dg (△) on force of contraction of guinea-pig isolated papillary muscles. The experimental procedure and the abbreviations used are the same as in Fig. 1 except that the incubation time of each concentration was 30 min. The pre-drug values were 1.40 ± 0.15 mN (n = 26).

Discussion

The present study shows that the hydrophilic polar metabolites of digitoxin and digoxin, digitoxin-16′-glucuronide and digoxin-16′-glucuronide, increase the force of contraction of ventricular muscle preparations isolated from human hearts. Roughly, the effects of the metabolites were similar to those obtained with the parent compounds digitoxin and digoxin. However, the metabolites tended to be slightly less potent than the parent compounds, but the differences were small (less than twofold) and were significant only in the case of digoxin. On the other hand, the maximal effects obtained with the metabolites were slightly greater than those of the parent compounds. This effect was especially pronounced in the case of digitoxin, albeit the difference was still insignificant. With respect to the time course, the build-up of the positive inotropic effects of all compounds required about 60 minutes. In contrast, the decline of the positive inotropic effect upon washing was about twice as fast in the case of the metabolites which is easily explained by the hydrophilic properties of these agents.

Similar results were obtained in papillary muscles isolated from guinea pigs. Again, the metabolites tended to be less potent and more effective than the parent compounds. However, it is noteworthy that digitoxin-16′-glucuronide was more than twice as effective as digitoxin in the guinea-pig papillary muscle. As in human hearts the decline of the positive inotropic effect upon washing was about twice as fast in the case of the hydrophilic metabolites.

In comparison with the results obtained by Belz and Heinz (1977) with digoxin-16′-glucuronide and digitoxin-16′-glucuronide in guinea-pig papillary muscles, the potency of the compounds was nearly identical. However, a greater efficacy was found in the present study. This is probably due to the fact that Belz and Heinz (1977) only allowed ten minutes for each concentration to produce its positive inotropic effect. This incubation period was obviously too short since the present study showed that approximately 60 min were required for reaching the maximum of the positive inotropic effects of these agents.

The question arises whether it is of any clinical significance that the glucuronides of digitoxin and digoxin produce distinct cardiotonic effects in the human heart. These metabolites are probably inappropriate to serve as new inotropic agents because of unfavourable pharmacokinetic properties. For instance, they are conceivably only poorly absorbed from the gastrointestinal tract and their elimination appears to be rapid (Petersen et al. 1977). They may, however, be clinically important in so far as they may contribute to the positive inotropic effects of the parent compounds and because they may cross-react with commonly used laboratory methods (^{86}Rb methods, radioimmunoassays) to determine the plasma levels of cardiac glycosides (Storstein et al. 1983).

References

1. Belz GG, Heinz N (1977) The influence of polar and non-polar digoxin and digitoxin metabolites on the ^{86}Rb-uptake of human erythrocytes and the contractility of guinea-pig papillary muscles. Arzneim-Forsch. (Drug Res) 27: 653–655
2. Lüllmann H, Peters T (1971) The cardioactivity of digitoxin metabolites. Eur J Pharmacol 14:204–205
3. Meinertz T, Nawrath H, Scholz H (1976) Possible role of cyclic AMP in the relaxation process of mammalian heart: Effects of dibutyryl cyclic AMP and theophylline on potassium contractures in cat papillary muscles. Naunyn Schmiedeberg's Arch Pharmacol 293:129–137
4. Petersen R, Flasch H, Heinz N (1977) Darstellung und Eigenschaften einiger Glukuronide und Sulfate von Cardenoliden und Cardenolid-glykosiden. Arzneim-Forsch. (Drug Res) 27:642–649
5. Rietbrock N, Woodcock RG (1981) Pharmacokinetics of digoxin and derivatives. In: Handbook of Experimental Pharmacology, Vol 56/II, Cardiac glycosides, Part II, Pharmacokinetics and clinical pharmacology (K. Greeff, ed), pp 31–56. (Springer, Berlin Heidelberg New York)
6. Storstein L (1981) Pharmacokinetics of digitoxin. In: Handbook of Experimental Pharmacology, Vol 56/II, Cardiac glycosides, Part II, Pharmacokinetics and clinical pharmacology (K. Greeff, ed), pp 3–30. Springer, Berlin, Heidelberg, New York
7. Storstein L, Scholz H, Oelert H, Flasch H, Schmitz W, Larsen A Clinical importance of conjugated digitoxin and digoxin metabolites in man. Submitted for publication 1983

Author's address:

Prof. Dr. Hasso Scholz, Abteilung Allgemeine Pharmakologie, Universitäts-Krankenhaus Eppendorf, Martinistraße 52, D-2000 Hamburg 20, (FRG)

Studies of the inotropic mechanisms of cardiac glycosides in cultured heart cells

Th. W. Smith, D. Kim and W. H. Barry

Cardiovascular Division, Brigham and Women's Hospital and Departments of Medicine, Brigham and Women's Hospital and Harvard Medical School, Boston, MA (USA)

Key words: digitalis, ouabain, NaK-ATPase, ion transport, inotropic effect

Extensive experimental work over the past several decades has explored virtually every mechanism known or suspected to modulate myocardial contractility in the search for the cellular basis of the positive inotropic effects of the cardiac glycosides (23). Recent investigative efforts have focused on mechanisms by which digitalis glycosides might enhance the availability of Ca^{++} to the myocardial contractile element, a final step in the inotropic process demonstrated by the elegant studies of Allen and Blinks using intracellular microinjection of the calcium-sensitive photoactive protein aequorin (2).

More than 20 years have passed since J. C. Skou first described the monovalent cation transport enzyme system, now known as NaK-ATPase, and Repke suggested the possibility that inhibition of this sarcolemmal enzyme by cardiac glycosides might underlie their positive inotropic effects (21). The very substantial evidence supporting NaK-ATPase as the receptor for the positive inotropic effects of the glycosides has been summarized in several recent reviews (1, 22, 23) and will not be reiterated in detail here. Generally lacking until quite recently, however, has been direct evidence establishing a causal link between glycoside-induced inotropy and inhibition of NaK-ATPase and hence of the active transport of Na^+ across the myocardial cell membrane. A central point of controversy has been the issue of whether significant Na^+ pump inhibition occurs at positively inotropic but subtoxic cardiac glycoside doses and plasma levels, or whether Na^+ pump inhibition is rather a late phenomenon leading to mechanical and/or electrophysiologic toxicity.

To address the latter issue, we studied an intact canine preparation in which ouabain was given by prolonged intravenous infusion after an initial loading dose (10). A sustained positive inotropic effect was achieved, with no rhythm disturbances or other evidence of toxicity even after 5 hours of continuous ouabain infusion. Serial left ventricular biopsies were obtained, and monovalent cation transport was studied *in vitro*. At times when an obvious positive intropic effect was evident (e.g., a 46% mean increase in maximum left ventricular dP/dt at 2 hours), inhibition of monovalent cation transport was invariably present when compared to biopsy samples from the same animal prior to ouabain administration. At 2 hours, uptake of the K^+ analog Rb^+ was reduced by a mean of 33%. Control animals given vehicle alone demonstrated no changes in myocardial contractile state or in monovalent cation active transport. In related studies, we found that subtoxic digoxin doses, producing a mean increase of 20% in LV maximum dP/dt, caused a 25% mean decrease in Rb^+ active uptake in LV biopsy samples, while toxic doses producing ventricular arrhythmias reduced Rb^+ active transport by 59% below control levels (11), with still greater inhibition to levels 80% below control at onset of fatal ventricular fibrillation with further digoxin infusion. Purkinje fiber monovalent cation transport was inhibited to a significantly greater extent than was found in simultaneously obtained myocardial samples at both subtoxic and toxic endpoints (24).

These studies, taken together, establish that a necessary condition is met in support of the hypothesis that Na^+ pump inhibition is causally related to a positive inotropic response to glycosides in an intact animal model. Because of reports from other laboratories (well summarized by Noble in reference 20) calling into question the role of Na^+ pump inhibition in cardiac glycoside-induced positive inotropy, we have also studied the effects of a broad range of ouabain concentrations in an isolated, electrically driven guinea pig left atrial preparation. These experiments were undertaken to address specifically the fact that cardiac glycosides at low concentrations in the 10^{-9} to 10^{-8}M range have been reported to produce no inhibition, or even a stimulation of monovalent cation active transport in isolated intact myocardium (20). Since digitalis is known to affect the release and metabolism of endogenous neurotransmitters that may influence inotropic state as well as NaK-ATPase activity and K^+ permeability, we also explored the interaction of low ouabain concentrations with adrenergic and cholinergic influences in isolated guinea pig left atrial preparations stimulated at 3.3 Hz. Inotropic state and monovalent cation transport (assessed by $^{86}Rb^+$ uptake) were measured simultaneously (15).

As we had found previously in quiescent atrial preparations (12), low concentrations of ouabain (10^{-9}M in these experiments) enhanced Rb^+ uptake by 25% with no concomitant change in contractile state; this stimulatory effect on transport was abolished either by propranolol or by atropine pretreatment. Atria pretreated with the muscarinic blocking agent atropine responded to 10^{-8}M ouabain with a small but significant positive inotropic effect (+10%), with no measureable inhibition of monovalent cation active transport. This positive inotropic response was abolished in atria from animals depleted of catecholamine stores by pretreatment with 6-hydroxydopamine, again suggesting a catecholamine dependence of the positive inotropic response of the isolated atrial preparation to ouabain concentrations in the 10^{-9} to 10^{-8}M range. At 10^{-7}M, ouabain always produced a positive inotropic response of about +25% independent of catecholamine depletion, beta adrenergic blockade, or muscarinic blockade. Inhibition of $^{86}Rb^+$ uptake accompanied the positive inotropic response only in the presence of propranolol. Under all circumstances studied, ouabain at concentrations above 10^{-7}M produced a positive inotropic response accompanied by significant inhibition of monovalent cation transport, while at concentrations 3×10^{-7}M and above, mechanical toxicity occurred except in those preparations pretreated with propranolol (15).

Even this brief description of our experimental findings in an intact tissue preparation will convey a sense of the complexity of the control of contractile state in myocardium with intact neurotransmitter stores and release mechanisms. Clearly, the mechanism as well as the magnitude of inotropic responses and Na^+ pump activity modulation are dependent on glycoside concentration. At low ouabain concentrations in the 1–10 nM range, inotropic and apparent monovalent cation transport responses of the left atrial preparation are mediated, at least in part, by effects on endogenous neurotransmitters. It must be emphasized, however, that the lack of correlation between inotropic effect and monovalent cation active transport as measured by $^{86}Rb^+$ uptake in the 10^{-9} to 10^{-7}M ouabain concentration range by no means excludes a key role of Na^+ pump inhibition in the inotropic mechanism of cardiac glycosides. As discussed by Eisner and colleagues (8) in correspondence related to the publication of Lechat *et al.* (15), one might expect Na^+ pump activity as measured by unidirectional K^+ or K^+ analog flux rates to return to baseline, albeit at a higher $[Na^+]_i$ level, in a preparation that had returned to a new steady state after inhibition of a sub-toxic fraction of Na^+ pump sites unless passive Na^+ entry had changed, the stoichiometry of the Na-K pump had changed, and/or unless some alternative pathway of Na^+ extrusion from the cell had become quantitatively more important.

Because of the extraordinary complexity of interpretation of experiments performed in intact myocardial preparations with their inherent diffusion limitations, uncertainties of interstitial space composition, and endogenous neuroeffector stores, we have chosen to pursue most of our studies of cardiac glycoside inotropic mechanism in preparations of spontaneously beating cultured heart cells from the chick embryo ventricle. This approach has a number of advantages for studies of basic cellular mechanisms, including 1) a substantial inotropic response to digitalis glycosides and the means to quantitate and record continuously that response; 2) rapid onset of stable inotropic responses to cardiac glycoside exposure, with prompt offset after drug washout; 3) methods to assess directly the effects of glycosides on unidirectional and net fluxes of Na^+, K^+ and Ca^{++} with good temporal resolution, and under conditions identical to those under which inotropic state is followed; 4) availability of means to resolve components of Ca^{++} fluxes in beating preparations under basal and glycoside-stimulated conditions; 5) availability of techniques to determine specific ouabain binding to NaK-ATPase sites using [^{3}H]ouabain, again under conditions identical to those used for assessment of contractile state; and 6) means to modulate the density of Na^+ pump sites in the intact, functioning cell. Descriptions of these methods may be found in the publications cited, and for the sake of brevity will not be reviewed here.

In an initial set of experiments, we established the time course and concentration-effect curve for the positive inotropic effect of ouabain and for the ouabain-induced inhibition of monovalent cation active transport (6). As shown in Figure 1, the positive inotropic effect of ouabain was well correlated with the extent of inhibition of $^{86}Rb^+$ uptake. The threshold for both phenomena is just above 10^{-7}M, and close correspondence is maintained up to 1.5×10^{-6}M, where toxicity began to emerge in this set of experiments. In parallel experiments, $[Na^+]_i$ was shown to be increased at concentrations of ouabain producing a positive inotropic effect, and these increases were accompanied by increases in a rapidly exchangeable intracellular Ca^{++} pool which we have studied subsequently in further detail (4) in experiments to define the kinetics of Ca^{++} exchange in the cultured heart cell preparation. The time course of Ca^{++} exchange can be resolved into two components. The rapid phase of exchange had a rate constant of 3.9 min^{-1} and accounted for roughly half of the total cellular Ca^{++} content. A slower exponential phase was identified that had a rate constant of 0.069 min^{-1}, and was fully labelled with $^{45}Ca^{++}$ by 120 min. Effects of the Ca^{++} channel-blocking drug verapamil and the trivalent Ca^{++} antagonist lanthanum on these Ca^{++} fluxes and pools were examined and confirm that the more rapidly exchangeable pool is closely related to contractile state (4).

Taken together, these studies support the hypothesis that Na^+ pump inhibition is causally related to the positive inotropic effect of glycosides in cultured chick embryo ventricular cells, but do not address directly the question of whether instantaneous Na^+ pump rate, cellular Na^+ content, or both are important in modulating Ca^{++} handling and contractile state. In further experiments to explore this issue, we studied the time course of return to baseline inotropic state after washout of ouabain and correlated it with recovery of monovalent cation transport rate and return toward normal of intracellular Na^+, K^+, and rapidly exchangeable Ca^{++} (3). Briefly stated, these studies showed that the return to baseline inotropic state was closely correlated with the return to control levels of monovalent cation transport rate and rapidly exchangeable cellular Ca^{++}, while $[Na^+]_i$ and $[K^+]_i$ values lagged behind and returned to normal later than did contractile state. Analogous observations of this sort of hysteresis have been noted by other workers using electrophysiologic techniques (9, 19) and suggest the possibility of a subsarcolemmal space within which Na^+ activity and Na^+–Ca^{++} exchange depend in a complex way on the transarcolemmal Na^+ efflux rate, the Na^+ influx rate, and the rate of exchange with bulk Na^+ in the intracellular pool.

The studies described thus far, together with findings of Lee and colleagues (17), Eisner and Lederer (7), Marban and Tsien (18), and Wasserstrom *et al.* (25), using electrophysiologic approaches, support the concept of a chain of events starting with binding of the cardiac glycoside to NaK-ATPase with consequent inhibition of monovalent cation transport and elevation of $[Na^+]_i$, leading to increased $[Ca^{++}]_i$ via enhanced Na^+–Ca^{++} exchange, as discussed in detail elsewhere (23). If this sequence correctly describes the basis for the positive inotropic effects of the glycosides, it should be possible to effect a similar response by other interventions that would specifically inhibit the Na^+ pump. A convenient means by which to reduce Na^+ pump activity is to decrease $[K^+]_o$. As predicted, reduction in $[K^+]_o$ from the normal level of 4 mM to 1 mM produced a positive inotropic response that was quite similar to that produced by 10^{-6}M ouabain or 5×10^{-5}M dihydroouabain.

If these three interventions all produce their inotropic effects by the sequence described above, the monovalent cation transport rate should be reduced and $[Na^+]_i$ should be increased to similar degrees in each instance. This indeed proved to be the case. $^{42}K^+$ uptake was reduced by 41% in response to 1.0 mM K^+, similar to the extent of inhibition achieved with the inotropically equipotent concentrations of ouabain and dihydroouabain (5). Increases in steady-state cellular Na^+ content were also very similar in response to glycosides or 1.0 mM K^+ (5).

The issue of Na^+–Ca^{++} exchange as a link in the chain of events leading to the positive inotropic effects of cardiac glycosides has been addressed more directly in recent experiments. We have schown that Ca^{++} influx in the cultured heart cell preparation is very sensitive to the transsarcolemmal Na^+ gradient, and can be augmented markedly by increases in $[Na^+]_i$ and/or by decreased $[Na^+]_o$ (4), as would be expected for Ca^{++} entry via Na^+–Ca^{++} exchange. We have performed experiments in which Ca^{++} influx was measured in response to a step change from normal to zero $[Na^+]_o$. Isotonicity was maintained by substitution of $[Na^+]_o$ with K^+, which depolarizes the cell and, in addition to zero $[Na^+]_o$, enhances the effect of any increase in $[Na^+]_i$ on Ca^{++} entry by Na^+–Ca^{++} exchange. At 10^{-7}M, ouabain caused no measureable change from baseline Ca^{++} entry, as would be expected from the findings summarized in Figure 1. At 2×10^{-7}M, however, ouabain caused both a positive inotropic response and stimulation of Na^+–Ca^{++} exchange (5), with both responses being more pronounced at 10^{-6}M ouabain. The time course of disappearance of the Ca^{++} influx stimulation after ouabain washout was also quite similar to the time course of dissipation of the positive inotropic effect (5).

Thus, the effects of cardiac glycosides on Na^+–Ca^{++} exchange are relatively easy to document under conditions such as zero $[Na^+]_o$ that augment the signal. Although the changes are less dramatic, we have also been able to demonstrate enhanced Ca^{++} influx and an increased rapidly exchangeable Ca^{++} pool in response to positively inotropic but subtoxic glycoside concentrations in the presence of normal $[Na^+]_o$ (5). While $[Ca^{++}]_i$ could very plausibly be increased in response to cardiac glycosides by a decrease in Ca^{++} efflux as well as by increased influx, our studies indicate that little Ca^{++} efflux occurs via Na^+–Ca^{++} exchange under physiologic conditions in the cultured chick embryo ventricular cell preparations and that the primary effect of the glycosides (at least at subtoxic concentrations) is to augment Ca^{++} entry (5). In support of this view, the stimulatory effect of 1 mM $[K^+]_o$ on Ca^{++} entry Na^+–Ca^{++} exchange was similar to that produced by equi-inotropic concentrations of glycosides (5).

We would emphasize that our results are not in conflict with the observations of Tsien and colleagues (18, 26) or Lederer and Eisner (16), who found an increase in slow inward Ca^{++} current in response to the increase in $[Ca^{++}]_i$ induced by Na^+ pump inhibition. This increase in slow inward current may well be an additional means by which cardiac glycosides augment contractile state, but as shown by Marban and Tsien (18), enhanced I_{si} is not a *necessary* condition for glycoside-induced inotropy to occur.

We have recently completed an additional series of experiments that provide further insight into the mechanism by which cardiac glycosides enhance contractile state in cultured heart

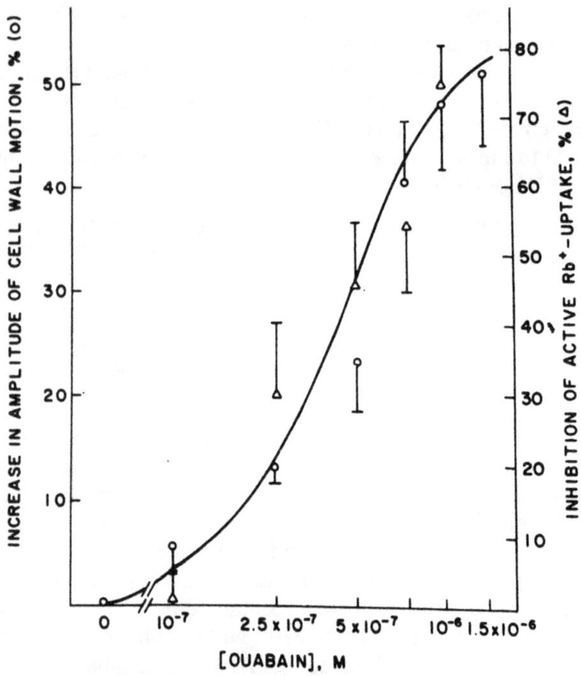

Fig. 1. Concentration-effect curve showing responses to ouabain of amplitude of cell wall motion (left scale) and inhibition of Rb^+ active transport (right scale). Points are means ± SEM of 4–14 experiments. The increase in contraction amplitude in percent shown the maximal effect at each ouabain concentration. Thresholds for significant inhibition of Rb^+ active transport and increase of contractility were between 10^{-7} and 2.5×10^{-7}M ouabain. The similar dependence of percent increase in amplitude of wall motion and percent inhibition of Rb^+ transport on ouabain concentration is evident. From Biedert *et al.* (6).

cells (13). Direct measurements of the specific binding of [^{3}H]ouabain to intact, beating cells yielded results indicating a single class of binding sites with a K_d in the absence of extracellular K^+ of 1.3×10^{-7}M. In the presence of 4 mM K^+, 10^{-7}M ouabain occupied 10% of the total number of binding sites and had no discernable effect on contractile state, active $^{42}K^+$ transport, or $[Na^+]_i$ (cf. Figure 1). A small but significant degree of Na-K pump inhibition could be demonstrated if cells were loaded with Na^+ in addition to being exposed to 10^{-7}M ouabain. At a concentration of 10^{-6}M ouabain, 38% of total specific ouabain binding sites were occupied and there was a significant increase in contractile amplitude within 30 seconds, reaching a plateau at about 7 min with a mean increase in contractile amplitude of 50%, a mean inhibition of the inward K^+ transport rate of 36%, and a 35% increase in $[Na^+]_i$ at steady state. Thus, the residual pool of unblocked Na^+ pump sites can maintain homeostasis by reaching a new steady state at which Na^+ efflux again equals Na^+ influx, but only with an increased $[Na^+]_i$ present to permit increased turnover of unblocked NaK-ATPase units. Indeed, the monovalent cation active transport rate could increase at least 4 times above baseline levels by preincubation in K^+-free medium to produce a substantial increase in $[Na^+]_i$. We conclude from these experiments that more than 10% of NaK-ATPase sites must be inhibited to produce measurable alterations in monovalent cation active transport, intracellular Na^+ content, or inotropic state. A positive inotropic effect is readily observed (together with increased $[Na^+]_i$ and Ca^{++} entry by Na^+–Ca^{++} exchange) when 36% of NaK-

ATPase units are blocked by ouabain, even though the reserve capacity of the Na^+ pump permits further increases in the turnover rate of unblocked sites in the presence of further elevations of $[Na^+]_i$.

Another approach to the assessment of the role of NaK-ATPase in the mechanism of inotropic action of digitalis glycosides that we have pursued recently is the growth of cultured heart cells under conditions such that increased numbers of NaK-ATPase sites are present in the sarcolemmal membrane. In this way, one should be able to distinguish between the validity of theories of digitalis action that postulate altered Ca^{++} binding to sarcolemmal sites as a result of glycoside interaction with NaK-ATPase and the mechanism proposed above – i.e., a positive inotropic effect that depends upon inhibition of the Na^+ pump and resulting increased levels of $[Na^+]_i$. In the former case, if the affinity of individual pump sites does not change, a larger number of NaK-ATPase complexes will result in more sites being occupied at a given ouabain concentration and should result in an enhanced inotropic response; if pump inhibition is requisite to the inotropic effect, then the greater number of unoccupied and functioning sites should render the cell less sensitive to both the inotropic and toxic effects of cardiac glycosides.

We were able to alter the pump site density in the sarcolemmal membrane by three different sets of growth conditions, each of which tended to increase steady-state $[Na^+]_i$: growth in a low K^+ concentration (1.0 mM), growth in a sublethal concentration of ouabain, or growth in 1 μM veratridine (14). These interventions produced increases of 60%, 40%, and 20% respectively in the total number of sites in the intact cell that specifically bound [^{3}H]ouabain. Acute exposure of control cells grown in 4.0 mM$[K^+]_o$ to 1.0 mM $[K^+]_o$ resulted in increases in $[Na^+]_i$ by an average of 37%, while after 48 hours of growth in 1.0 mM $[K^+]_o$, $[Na^+]_i$ declined to near-baseline values. Thus the increased density of [^{3}H]ouabain binding sites represented a pool of functional Na^+ pumps; binding studies over a range of [^{3}H]ouabain concentrations yielded Scatchard plots showing that the increase in B_{max} was not accompanied by any change in binding site affinity, which continued to represent a single population of sites as judged by the linearity of the Scatchard plots. The intrinsic contractile responsiveness of the populations of cells with enhanced numbers of NaK-ATPase sites to the β-adrenergic agonist isoproterenol was unchanged from control levels.

In contrast to the unchanged isoproterenol responsiveness, cells grown in low K^+ with increased numbers of Na^+ pump sites were clearly hyporesponsive to ouabain. The ouabain concentration-effect curve for positive inotropy underwent a parallel shift to the right (to higher ouabain concentrations). Accompanying this change was a rapid component of Ca^{++} uptake in response to a step change in $[Na^+]_o$ from normal to zero (interpreted as Ca^{++} entry by Na^+–Ca^{++} exchange) that was significantly lower in the low K^+-grown cells than in control cells equilibrated for just 30 minutes in 1.0 mM $[K^+]_o$. This blunted contractile response to ouabain of cells with augmented numbers of Na^+ pump sites is consistent with the view that elevated $[Na^+]_i$, due to inhibition of NaK-ATPase, is requisite to the positive inotropic effects of cardiac glycosides, probably involving a subsequent step of enhanced Na^+–Ca^{++} exchange across the sarcolemma. Our results further argue against altered membrane Ca^{++} binding properties, as opposed to pump inhibition *per se,* as the basis of the inotropic response.

This description of experimental results in our studies using cultured heart cells illustrates, we believe, several of the advantages of this system in the dissection of fundamental aspects of the modulation of contractile state. While these findings provide a plausible basis on which to build hypotheses, it remains for future studies to provide definitive experimental evidence regarding the mechanism or mechanisms by which cardiac glycosides enhance contractile state in the *in situ* heart of the intact animal, and ultimately to understand in detail the cellular basis for the effects of digitalis as observed in clinical use.

References

1. Akera T, Brody TM (1978) The role of Na^+, K^+-ATPase in the inotropic action of digitalis. Pharmacol Rev 29:187–220
2. Allen DG, Blinks JR (1978) Calcium transients in aequorin-injected frog cardiac muscle. Nature (London) 273:509–513
3. Barry WH, Biedert S, Miura DS, Smith TW (1981) Changes in cellular Na, K, and Ca contents, monovalent cation transport rate, and contractile state during washout of cardiac glycosides from cultured chick heart cells. Circ Res 49:141–149
4. Barry WH, Smith TW (1982) Mechanisms of transmembrane calcium movement in cultured chick embryo ventricular cells. J Physiol (London) 325: 243–260
5. Barry WH, Hasin Y, Smith TW Sodium pump inhibition, enhanced Ca influx via Na-Ca exchange, and positive inotropic response in cultured heart cells (Submitted)
6. Biedert S, Barry WH, Smith TW (1979) Inotropic effects and changes in sodium and calcium contents associated with inhibition of monovalent cation active transport by ouabain in cultured myocardial cells. J Gen Physiol 74:479–494.
7. Eisner DA, Lederer WJ (1979) Does sodium pump inhibition produce the positive inotropic effects of strophanthidin in mammalian cardiac muscle? J Physiol (London) 296):75P–76P
8. Eisner DA, Vaughan-Jones RD, Lederer WJ (1983) Comments on "Active transport and inotropic state in guinea pig left atrium". Circ Res 53:834–835
9. Ellis D (1977) The effects of external cations and ouabain on the intracellular sodium activity of sheep heart purkinje fibers. J Physiol (London) 273:211–240
10. Hougen TJ, Smith TW (1978) Inhibition of myocardial monovalent cation active transport by subtoxic doses of ouabain in the dog. Circ Res 42:856–863
11. Hougen TJ, Lloyd BL, Smith TW (1979) Effects of inotropic and arrhythmogenic digoxin doses and of digoxin-specific antibody on myocardial monovalent cation transport in the dog. Circ Res 44: 23–31
12. Hougen TJ, Spicer N, Smith TW (1981) Stimulation of myocardial cation active transport by low concentrations of cardiac glycosides: Role of catecholamines. J Clin Invest 48:1207–1214
13. Kim D, Barry WH, Smith TW Unpublished data.
14. Kim D, Marsh JD, Barry WH, Smith TW Effects of growth in low K^+ medium or ouabain on membrane NaK-ATPase, cation transport and contractility in cultured chick heart cells. Circ Res (in press)
15. Lechat P, Malloy CR, Smith TW (1983) Active transport and inotropic state in guinea pig left atrium. Circ Res 52:411–422
16. Lederer WJ, Eisner DA (1982) The effects of sodium pump activity on the slow inward current in sheep cardiac purkinje fibers. Proc R Soc London Ser B 214:249–262
17. Lee CO, Kang DH, Sokol JH, Lee KS (1980) Relation between intracellular Na ion acitivity and tension of sheep cardiac purkinje fibers exposed to dihydro-ouabain. Biophys J 29:315–330
18. Marban E, Tsien RW (1982) Enhancement of calcium current during digitalis inotropy in mammalian heart – positive feed-back by intracellular calcium? J Physiol (London) 329:589–614
19. Miura DS, Rosen MR (1978) The effects of ouabain on the transmembrane potentials and intracellular potassium activity of canine cardiac purkinje fibers. Circ Res 42:333–338
20. Noble D (1980) Mechanism of action of therapeutic levels of cardiac glycosides. Cardiovasc Res 14:495–514
21. Repke K (1962) Metabolism of cardiac glycosides. Proc Pharmacol Meet 1st, Vol 3, p 47
22. Schwartz A, Lindenmayer GE, Allen JC (1975) The sodium-potassium adenosine triphosphatase: Pharmacological, physiological and biochemical aspects. Pharmacol Rev 27:3–134
23. Smith TW, Barry WH (1983) Monovalent cation transport and mechanisms of digitalis-induced inotropy. In: Current Topics In Membranes And Transport 19:857–884. J. Hoffman and B. Forbush, (Eds)
24. Somberg JC, Barry WH, Smith TW (1981) Differing sensitivities of purkinje fibers and myocardium to inhibition of monovalent cation transport by digitalis. J Clin Invest 67:116–123
25. Wasserstrom JA, Schwartz DJ, Fozzard HA (1983) Relation between intracellular sodium and twitch tension in sheep cardiac purkinje strands exposed to cardiac glycosides. Circ Res 521:697–705
26. Weingart R, Kass RS, Tsien RW (1981) Is digitalis inotropy associated with enhanced slow inward calcium current? Nature (London) 273:389–392

Authors' address:

Dr. Th. W. Smith, Cardiovascular Div., Brigham and Women's Hospital, Boston, MA 02115 (USA)

Therapeutic range of cardiac glycosides

K.-O. Haustein

Section of Clinical Pharmacology of the Institute of Pharmacology and Toxicology of the Medical Academy Erfurt, Erfurt (GDR)

Summary

The narrow therapeutic range of cardiac glycosides continually challenges chemists to synthetize new derivatives with improved therapeutic properties. One of the best investigated semi-synthetic glycosides is 16α-gitoxin. Compared to ouabain and gitoxin, it produces positive inotropic effects on the isolated guinea-pig heart in a wider range of concentrations and causes less pronounced rhythmic disturbances. These results were confirmed by electrophysiological investigations in isolated fibres of the canine myocardium and of the Purkinje system, by investigations in the anaesthetized cat and dog and in healthy volunteers. The effects of various semi-synthetic compounds (e.g. actodigin, ASI-222) are described and possibilities to trigger these effects are discussed. Of some significance seem to be differences in the structure of the $(Na^+ + K^+)$-ATPase system of different tissues, e.g. the working muscle and the Purkinje system of the heart, as well as differences due to the formation and dissociation of the glycoside-enzyme complex. The significance of K^+,Ca^{2+} and of several pharmacokinetic parameters (e.g. the volume of distribution) for these reactions are briefly discussed.

Key words: Cardiac glycosides, 16α-gitoxin, actodigoxin, therapeutic range, systolic time intervals

Introduction

The narrow difference between the therapeutic range and toxic dose of the naturally occurring, therapeutically used cardioactive glycosides is a general problem which has not yet been solved. Since the report of Neumann (24) many attempts have been made to alter the structure of naturally occurring cardiotonic steroids using semi-synthetic procedures. In the past 20 years many glycosides have been synthetized and most of them have the modification in the sugar moiety. These steroids were synthetized with the aim of improving the therapeutic properties, e.g. the absorption from the gastrointestinal tract. Many cardiotonic steroids with changes in the sugar moiety have a high percentage of absorption without improved therapeutic range (cf. 7). In contrast to these findings, Battermann et al. (1) described a better therapeutic range of gitalin. They found that the therapeutic dose amounts to nearly 40 per cent of toxic dose whereas that of digitoxin amounts to 60 per cent. Several authors confirmed these results (32), whereas they were in contradiction to those of other workers (11, 18, 30).

16α-gitoxin – The first cardioactive glycoside with improved therapeutic range

A striking success was the synthesis of 16α-gitoxin by Lindig and coworkers (21). In contrast to the most changes in cardiotonic steroids, the variation of structure was inserted in the genin moiety.

Following the results of Repke and coworkers (27), the inhibitory curve of 16α-gitoxin shows an extraordinarily flat slope within the therapeutically effective range of concentrations in contrast to that of ouabain and the other naturally occurring cardiotonic steroids. This slow rise of the curve can be seen up to about 30 per cent inhibition of the enzyme after which the curve follows the usual slope. This prompted us to carry out several animal experiments.

We investigated 16α-gitoxin in the isolated, spontaneously beating atrium and in the spontaneously beating, perfused heart of the guinea-pig. For measurement of the positive as well as negative inotropic effect with the glycoside, we used ΔI_t as a measure of the extent and duration of the effect because these inotropic effects vary with time of exposure and concentration (5). We assessed the occurrence of arrhythmias and calculated the mean arrhythmia percentage throughout the test period (A_t). The results obtained in the isolated heart corroborated our hypothesis of the enhanced therapeutic margin of 16α-gitoxin. 16α-gitoxin, gitoxin and ouabain, when applied in equieffective concentrations, attained their maximum positive inotropic effects at almost the same rate (K^+ concentration 2.56 mMol.l^{-1}). However, the extent and duration of the effects differed considerably and were dependent on the nature and concentration of the glycoside. To increase the ΔI_t-values from 5 per cent to maximum, the bath concentrations of the glycosides had to be raised by factors 4.0 (ouabain), 5.5 (gitoxin) and 24.0 (16α-gitoxin). Thus, the range of concentrations improving contractility was clearly greater with 16α-gitoxin (Fig. 1) (17).

In the isolated guinea-pig heart perfused with constant glycoside concentrations, ouabain and 16α-gitoxin developed positive inotropic effects more slowly than gitoxin, but they lasted for a prolonged period of time. A comparison of the glycoside concentrations required to produce maximum ΔI_t-values in isolated hearts showed that the relative inotropic efficacy of 16α-gitoxin was greater in isolated hearts than in the atria while the opposite was true for ouabain and gitoxin. Since the tension developed by the isolated hearts was due mainly to the ventricular muscle, the results strongly suggest that the action of 16α-gitoxin extends preferentially to the ventricle. A decrease in ΔI_t was observed with glycoside perfusion at higher concentrations than those required to produce maximum values of ΔI_t. This effect was mainly due to ventricular tachycardia and fibrillation, although some arrhythmias occurred before ΔI_t had reached its maximum, particularly with ouabain and gitoxin. Thus, an increase in ΔI_t from 10 to 40 per cent raised the frequency of arrhythmias from 10 to 70 per cent (ouabain), from 45 to 100 per cent (gitoxin) and from 0 to 10 per cent (16α-gitoxin) (17).

In experiments with three different potassium concentrations in the nutritive medium, distinct differences in the properties of the 3 glycosides were observed (Fig. 1). At 1.34

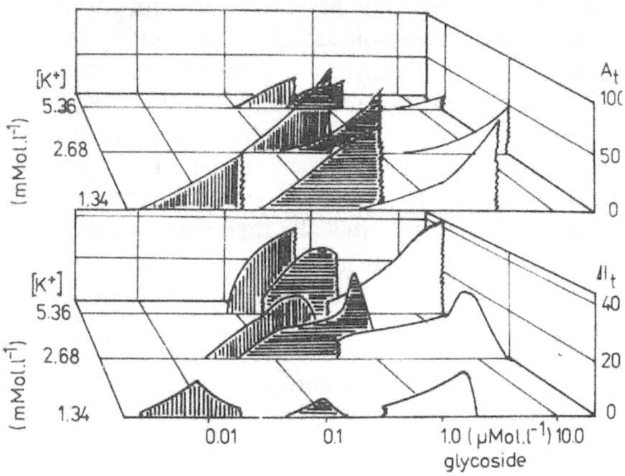

Fig. 1. Actions of ouabain, gitoxin and 16α-gitoxin on the contractility (lower part) and arrhythmia percentage (upper part) of spontaneously beating atria of guinea-pig heart at 1.34, 2.68 and 5.36 mMol.l^{-1} $[K^+]_o$.
Ouabain: vertically lined areas, gitoxin: horizontally lined areas, 16α-gitoxin: open areas. The broken line at the right side of the areas demonstrate that the following glycoside concentration (factor = $\sqrt{2}$) gives toxicity (negative inotropic effects) (12)

$mMol.l^{-1}$ $[K^+]_o$, ouabain, gitoxin and 16α-gitoxin enhanced the contractile force of the atria only slightly, whereas there was a high frequency of arrhythmias. The three glycosides behaved similarly. The range of concentrations in which the glycosides mainly increase contractility is rather small and thus, the therapeutic ranges overlap. If $[K^+]_o$ was enhanced to 5.36 $mMol.l^{-1}$, the maximum increment of contractility was increased and arrhythmias infrequently occurred (12, 14).

With regard to a faster poisoning of Purkinje fibres than of ventricular fibres of the canine heart by ouabain (30), the effects of a glycoside with improved therapeutic range seemed of special interest. Glycoside concentrations causing a distinct increase in contractile force (0.125 $\mu Mol.l^{-1}$ ouabain, 2.5 $\mu Mol.l^{-1}$ 16α-gitoxin) in the isolated guinea-pig heart, showed no differences in toxic effects in canine hearts (cf. Table 1). Both glycoside concentrations showed the same time course of poisoning of ventricular muscle fibres while marked differences were observed in the time course of poisoning of the Purkinje fibres. Fibres exposed to both low glycoside concentrations had 2.5 times higher survival time after 16α-gitoxin than after ouabain (25). Thus, the wide therapeutic range of 16α-gitoxin is based on the weak effect on the specialized conducting system.

Table 1. Survival time of isolated ventricular and Purkinje fibres of the canine heart after glycoside infusion (25)

Glycoside	Concentration (μmol^{-1})	Survival time (min ± S.D.) Ventricular muscle fibres	Purkinje fibres
16α-Gitoxin	1.5	343 ± 62 (4)	200 ± 49 (5)$^{\times}$
	2.5	156 ± 21 (4)	68 ± 3 (3)
Ouabain	0.1	321 ± 57 (4)	81 ± 11 (5)$^{\times}$
	0.125	186 ± 31 (4)	89 ± 21 (5)

$^{\times}$ The two values marked differ significantly ($p < 0.001$); number of experiments indicated in parentheses

The results of the infusion experiments in cats showed that lethal effects occurred at both ouabain infusion rates after nearly identical total doses (13). 16α-gitoxin exerted its lethal effects dependent on the infusion rate at different total doses (cf. Table 2). At the low 16α-gitoxin infusion rate, less glycoside amounts would be required for lethal effects, provided that glycoside elimination through the kidneys is slow. The occurrence of ECG changes (prolongation of QRS) after 89 per cent only of the lethal dose of 16α-gitoxin represents an exception among glycoside effects in general. This effect of 16α-gitoxin is in accordance with the results obtained in the dog (13). In the case of ouabain concentrations, no differences existed between lethal doses and doses producing prolongation of the QRS complex (cf. Table 2). This effect might be explained as an "over-titration effect" operative in the more glycoside-sensitive conductive system only (31).

In addition, investigations were carried out in healthy volunteers. The i.v. injection of 5 or 7.5 mg 16α-gitoxin within 15 min provoked a maximum shortening of the systolic time intervals $LVET_c$ and QS_{2c}. A second maximum was reached after 1.5 h, and after 4 h a minimum was observed (Figure 2B). Calculating the AUC-values (0–2 h) of the effects depending on the dose, a linear regression line was obtained (Figure 2A) as was the case with digitoxin and digoxin (2) and with 16-acetyl-gitoxin (16). In spite of the inotropic maximum (15 ms in case of $\Delta LVET_c$ and 25 ms in case of ΔQS_{2c}) the mean PQ-time intervals of the ECG

Table 2. Prolongation of QRS complex producing and lethal doses of 16α-gitoxin and ouabain in anaesthetized cats (13)

Glycoside	n	Infusion rate ($nmol.kg^{-1}.min^{-1}$)	Glycoside dose ($mg.kg^{-1}$) QRS prolongation$^{\times}$	Infused up to cardiac arrest
16α-Gitoxin	8	100.0	3.83 ± 0.51	5.64 ± 0.63
	7	200.0	3.98 ± 0.64	4.47 ± 0.99
Ouabain	7	5.0	0.059 ± 0.017	0.12 ± 0.024
	6	10.0	0.092 ± 0.028	0.14 ± 0.012

$^{\times}$ QRS complex > 0.03 sec

and the heart rate decreased only slightly, while the QT_c-intervals of the ECG were abbreviated distinctly (Figure 2B).

Position of 16α-gitoxin among naturally occurring glycosides

The differences in the therapeutic range of naturally occurring glycosides and of 16α-gitoxin can be explained mainly by different actions on the working muscle of the heart and the Purkinje system. When applied to the molecular level, differences in the affinity of the glycosides for various $(Na^+ + K^+)$-ATPase systems are supposed. Such differences are well-known in ATPase systems of various tissues, e.g. of the heart muscle and the brain from different animals and the human being (Table 3) (19, 27). The temporary differences in the occurrence of the glycoside effect could be also explained by the results obtained in studying the kinetic parameters of the enzyme system (28). Accordingly, the delayed onset of Purkinje fibre inexcitability following 16α-gitoxin could be due to a much higher dissociation rate of the glycoside-receptor complex. In the membrane ATPase system of the guinea-pig heart, binding constants for formation of glycoside-receptor complexes vary only slightly, whereas the dissociation of the complex was 30 times faster in the case of 16α-gitoxin than in the case of

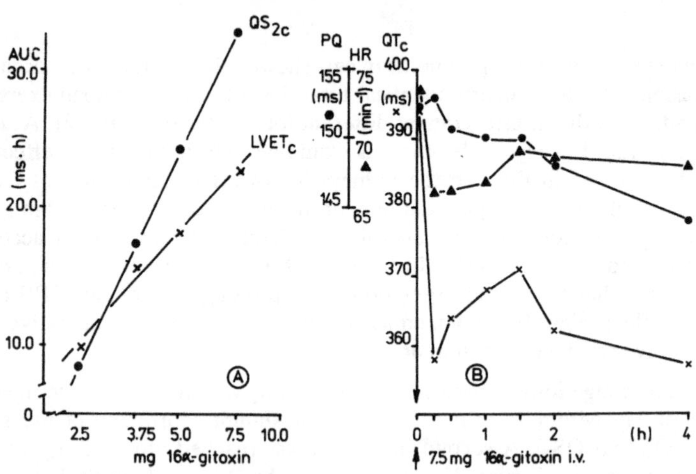

Fig. 2. The effects of 16α-gitoxin on systolic time intervals $LVET_c$ and QS_{2c} (A; AUC^2 in ms.h) after i.v. injection of 2.5, 3.75, 5.0 and 7.5 mg in healthy volunteers, and time course of QT_c and PQ-interval of the ECG and heart rate after i.v. injection of 7.5 mg 16α-gitoxin in 6 healthy volunteers (B).

Table 3. Therapeutic properties of naturally occurring and semi-synthetic cardioactive steroids (Data calculated from the results of the authors, activity of ouabain = 1.0)

Glycoside	A/I	L/I	Method	Authors
Ouabain	1.0	1.0	canine heart-lung preparation	Imai et al. (20)
Peruvoside	2.0	1.5		
Proscillaridin A	0.4	0.3		
Ouabain	1.0	1.0	anaesthetized dog	Caldwell and Nash (4)
ASI-222	2.9	3.1		
Ouabain	1.0	1.0	anaesthetized dog	Mendez et al. (23)
Dihydro-ouabain	1.8	1.7		
Actodigin	2.1	2.8		
Ouabain	1.0	1.0	guinea-pig atrium	Haustein et al. (17)
16α-Gitoxin	1.2	1.3		

A/I: arrhythmogenic to inotropic dose, L/I: lethal to inotropic dose

ouabain (28). We suppose that the glycoside binding receptor areas of the membrane ATPase system of Purkinje and ventricular muscle fibres vary in conformation and possibly in structure. Differences in kinetics between the appearance of the effect and its disappearance or between complex formation and dissociation could be due to different glycoside-binding receptors. In general, we believe that close correlation exists between the exceptional effects of 16α-gitoxin on the isolated heart and the flat slope of the concentration-dependent inhibition of the enzyme.

Other cardioactive glycosides with improved therapeutic range

Within the past years several authors published analoguous conceptions of the existence of glycosides with a comparatively high margin of safety. Among a great number of compounds the following must be mentioned: actodigin (AY-22,241) (23, 26), ASI-222 (4, 6), and α-methyl-digitoxigenin glucoside (22). Acetyl-strophanthidin was of secondary interest (8–10). Most compounds were investigated with analogous methods. In comparison to ouabain, quotients of these steroids between lethal to inotropic and lethal to arrhythmogenic dose were enhanced (cf. Table 4). Besides the mentioned semi-synthetic compounds, the naturally occurring glycosides peruvoside and proscillaridin A were included in the investigations (20). In contrast to the compounds tested which are monosides, 16α-gitoxin is a tridigitoxoside as are digitoxin and digoxin. As all the new compounds tested, 16α-gitoxin exerts its cardiotonic effects in vitro and in vivo in 10 to 20fold higher concentrations or doses than the naturally occurring glycosides. Actodigin has a rapid onset of cardiac action as 16α-gitoxin and acetyl-strophanthidin. 16α-gitoxin is superior to the strophanthidin derivative in that it lacks arrhythmogenic effects (8, 10, 29) and also to actodigin in that it does not give early ventricular arrhythmias in the anaesthetized cat. Actodigin causes a marked decrease in heart rate and a profound prolongation of the PR-interval possibly due to a greater increase in vagal tone than observed in case of 16α-gitoxin (3). These in vivo results are in contradiction to those obtained in vitro by Pastelin and Mendez (26). In comparison to actodigin, the onset of action of 16α-gitoxin is rapid and the action of actodigin disappears possibly as fast as that of 16α-gitoxin (13, 23).

General conclusions

The results obtained with 16α-gitoxin and those of the literature (most of all concerning actodigin) allow the following statements: (1) Cardioactive steroids with a high margin of

Table 4. Inhibition of the $(Na^{+}+K^{+})$-ATPase system from human heart and brain by digitoxin and digoxin (IC_{50} in $\mu mol.l^{-1}$. Mean ± S.D.) (19)

Glycoside	Heart	Brain
Digitoxin	0.124 ± 0.040	0.215 ± 0.046
Digoxin	0.075 ± 0.018	0.185 ± 0.020

safety are positive inotropically effective in a wide range of concentrations. (2) With these glycosides, the Purkinje system is affected to a lesser extent than by naturally occurring glycosides (e.g. ouabain) and toxic reactions disappear due to reversible effects (wash-out). Up to now it is unclear whether these differences in action are caused by differences in the kinetics on the molecular level (glycoside-enzyme complex) or by differences on the tissue level (e.g. distribution of the glycoside between myocardium and Purkinje system). (3) The known glycosides with a comparatively great margin of safety act in 10 to 20fold higher doses or concentrations than naturally occurring glycosides, possibly on the basis of changed kinetics on the drug-enzyme level (formation and dissociation of the glycoside-enzyme complex). (4) It is not yet clear whether the pharmacokinetics of the semi-synthetic glycosides contribute to the improved therapeutic range. In experiments with continuous infusion of the glycoside its properties such as distribution rate and volume of distribution are neglected. (5) The effects of a glycoside on contractility and rhythmicity can be changed by variation of $[K^{+}]$ and $[Ca^{2+}]$ in the nutritive medium, that means the reaction of the glycosides is possibly subjected to different K^{+}- and Ca^{2+}-fluxes during and after excitation in myocardium and conducting system.

References

1. Battermann RC, de Graff AC, Rose OE (1952) Therapeutic range of gitalin (amorphous) compared with other digitalis preparations. Circulation 5:201–207
2. Belz GG, Erbel R, Schumann K, Gilfrich HJ (1978) Dose-response relationships and plasma concentrations of digitalis glycosides in man. Eur J clin Pharm 13:103–111
3. Cagin NA, Somberg J, Bounous H, Levitt B (1977) A comparison of actodigin and ouabain in cats. Arch int Pharmacodyn 226:263–269
4. Caldwell RW, Nash CB (1976) Pharmacological studies of a new 4-aminosugar cardiac glycoside (ASI-222). J Pharm Exptl Ther 197:19–26
5. Caprio A, Farah A (1967) The effect of the isotonic milieu on the response of rabbit cardiac muscle to ouabain. J Pharm Exptl Ther 155:403–414
6. Cook LS, Caldwell RW, Nash CB (1977) Comparison of the cardiac effects of ASI-222 HCl, an aminosugar cardiac glycoside and digoxin. Arch int Pharmacodyn 227:220–232
7. Diederen W, Kadatz R (1970) Quantitative Untersuchungen der therapeutischen Breite von Herzglykosiden. Ärztl Forsch 24:149–155
8. Enselberg CD, Croce JP, Lown B (1951) Ventricular fibrillation due to digitalis preparations. Circulation 3:647–657
9. Gold H, Modell W, Kwitt NT, Shane SJ, Dayrit G, Kramer ML, Zahm W, Otto HL (1948) Comparison of ouabain with strophanthidin-3-acetate by intravenous injection in man. J Pharmac Exptl Ther 94:39–43
10. Gold H, Otto HL, Modell W, Halpern SL (1947) Behaviour of synthetic esters of strophanthidin, the acetate, propionate, butyrate, and benzoate in man. J Pharmac Exptl Ther 86:301–309
11. Gruhzit CC, Farah AE (1953) Determination of the therapeutic range of gitalin in the heart-lung preparation of the dog. J Pharmac Exptl Ther 108:113–116
12. Haustein K-O (1973) Comparison of therapeutic and toxic actions of ouabain, gitoxin and 16-epigitoxin on isolated atria at different extracellular potassium concentrations. Europ J Pharmac 21:195–202

13. Haustein K-O (1977) Extraordinary cardiac effects of 16-epi-gitoxin in comparison to ouabain in cats and dogs. Pharmacology (Basel) 15:178–190
14. Haustein K-O, Graumann G, Stephan B (1975) Studies on cardioactive steroids – III. Characterization of different cardiac glycosides by their effects of contractility and rhythmicity at different extracellular potassium concentrations. Acta biol med germ 34:1065–1073
15. Haustein K-O, Hauptmann J (1974) Studies on cardioactive steroids – II. Structure-activity relationships in the isolated guinea-pig heart. Pharmacology (Basel) 11:127–138
16. Haustein K-O, Hentschel H Über die dosisabhängige Verkürzung der systolischen Zeitintervalle nach Einnahme von Pengitoxin. Arzneimittel-Forsch (Drug Res) in press
17. Haustein K-O, Markwardt F, Repke KRH (1970) Different relationships between therapeutic and toxic actions of 16-epi-gitoxin, gitoxin and ouabain on isolated cardiac preparations. Eur J Pharmac 10:1–10
18. Hejtmancik MR, Herrmann GR (1952) A clinical study of gitalin. Arch int Med 90:224–233
19. Hentschel C, Haustein K-O Zur Wirkung von 16-Acetyl-gitoxin auf das ($Na^{+}+K^{+}$)-ATPase-System des menschlichen Herzens und Gehirns. Arzneimittel-Forsch (Drug Res) (in press)
20. Imai S, Katano Y, Takeda K, Kumada M, Iizuka H, Shiraki Y, Sakai K (1972) A quantitative comparison of the cardiac actions of peruvoside with those of g-strophanthidin and proscillaridin. Tohoku J exp Med 108:389–399
21. Lindig C, Megges R, Repke K (1966) 16-Epi-gitoxin, ein neues partialsynthetisches Herzglykosid. Naunyn-Schmiedeberg's Arch exp Path Pharmak 253:66–67
22. Lüllmann H, Peters T, Ziegler A (1979) Kinetic events determining the effects of cardiac glycosides. Trends Pharmac Sci 1:102–106
23. Mendez R, Pastelin G, Kabela E (1974) The influence of the position of the attachment of the lactone ring to the steroid nucleus on the action of cardiac glycosides. J Pharmac Exptl Ther 188:189–197
24. Neumann W (1937) Vergleichende Untersuchungen über die pharmakokinetische Wirksamkeit von natürlichen und synthetischen Derivaten des k-Strophanthidins. Naunyn-Schmiedeberg's Arch Path Pharmak 185:329–352
25. Nowak G, Haustein K-O (1976) Different toxic effects of ouabain and 16-epi-gitoxin on Purkinje-fibres and ventricular muscle fibres. Pharmacology (Basel) 14:256–264
26. Pastelin G, Mendez R (1972) Singular effects of a new short acting glycoside in Purkinje cells. Eur J Pharmac 19:291–293
27. Repke K, Est M, Portius HJ (1965) Über die Ursache der Speziesunterschiede in der Digitalisempfindlichkeit. Biochem Pharmac 14:1785–1802
28. Repke KRH, Herrmann I, Kunze R, Portius HJ, Schön R, Schönfeld W Mechanisms of digitalis action and the importance of the kinetics of the formation and decomposition of glycoside-receptor complex for understanding of overall pharmacokinetics of digitalis compounds. In: Symposium on Digitalis, pp. 143–151, Storstein O (Ed.) Gyldendal Norsk Forlag, Oslo 1973
29. Sarnoff SJ, Gilmore JP, Mitchell HJ, Remensnyder JP (1963) Potassium changes in the heart during homeostatic autoregulation and acetyl strophanthidin. Am J Med 34:440–451
30. Schwiegk H (1960) Die Therapie der Herzinsuffizienz mit Glykosiden. Internist (Berlin-W.) 1:6–14
31. Vassalle M, Karis J, Hoffman BF (1962) Toxic effects of ouabain on Purkinje fibres and ventricular muscle fibres. Am J Physiol 203:433–439
32. Weiss A, Steigmann F (1954) Gitalin in the treatment of congestive heart failure: a clinical study. Am J Med 227:188–192

Author's address:

Prof. Dr. K.-O. Haustein, Section of Clinical Pharmacology, Institute of Pharmacology and Toxicology of the Medical Academy Erfurt, Nordhäuser Str. 74, GDR-5010 Erfurt

Increased therapeutic range, merely a pharmacokinetic problem?

K. Kochsiek

Department of Medicine, University Hospital "Luitpoldkrankenhaus", Würzburg (FRG)

Key words: Cardiac glycosides, pharmaco-kinetics, serum levels, myocardial glycoside concentration, toxicity

The difficulty with this topic begins already with the definition of the term "therapeutic range". In the clinic the limits of the therapeutic range are determined by the dose of a drug necessary for a therapeutic effect and the dose at which toxic effects begin. For digitalis glycosides the therapeutic range lies between the amount of drug required for the beginning of positive inotropic effects and that amount at which toxic side effects (generally arrhythmias) are caused. Here difficulties appear already since at present no methods exist for the definite recognition of the onset of positive inotropic effects. A few weeks ago, a symposium was held on the theme of "Evaluation of Methods for the Measurement of Inotropic Effects". The conclusion of the workshop discussion was that there are no clinically reliable or sufficiently sensitive methods for the measurement of inotropic changes*. Even in experimental pharmacology the determination of the therapeutic range of digitalis glycosides is problematic. Many experimental investigators using i.v. infusions have defined the therapeutic range as the dose range between onset of arrhythmias and the lethal dose (1). However, this definition does not satisfy practical requirements and for understandable reasons cannot be applied to clinical situations. The onset of the arrhythmic effects of glycosides approximately corresponds to the maximal rather than the minimal increase in inotropy. From the clinical standpoint, the therapeutic range lies between the doses causing minimal and maximal inotropic effects, not between the doses causing arrhythmic and lethal effects, since the latter two effects are both toxic ones which should be avoided in the clinical setting. However, a few investigators measured the dose causing positive inotropic effects and arrhythmic and lethal effects during continuous i.v. infusion. Even this experimental model cannot be compared to the clinical situation since glycosides are usually given orally in the clinic, with the use of increasing doses for initial digitalization, or a constant dose in maintenance therapy.

Using sensitive assays for serum glycoside levels, it was concluded that the desired therapeutic effect, or the toxic effects, were more a function of the serum glycoside level than the dose of glycoside given, although, on the average, a linear correlation has been shown between the oral maintenance dose and serum glycoside levels in large collective studies (16).

The close correlation between serum glycoside levels and effects suggests a linear correlation between serum level and glycoside concentration in heart muscle. The concentration of digoxin or β-methyldigoxin in left ventricular papillary muscle and in serum is shown in figure 1. Papillary muscle was obtained post mortem at autopsy, and the serum sample was obtained shortly before death (12). The correlation between serum and tissue glycoside level was even closer when samples were simultaneously obtained, as for example during cardiac surgery. The correlation between the glycoside concentrations simultaneously determined in serum and in operatively resected papillary muscle is shown in figure 2. Compared to fig. 1, a better correlation is seen. The eleven patients labelled "R" developed various forms of arrhythmias in the immediate postoperative phase. The serum glycoside level of this group

*"Bewertung von Methoden zur Inotropiemessung", Ulm Oct. 6th, 1983 (non published)

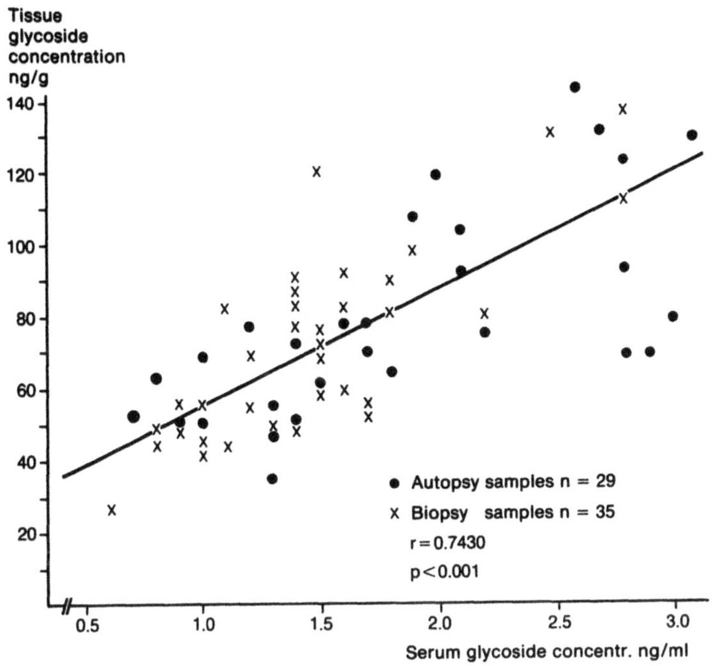

Fig. 1. Correlation between glycoside concentration in serum and left ventricular papillary muscle from biopsy and autopsy material taken from 64 patients (17)*.

was 1.8 ± 0.46 ng/ml which was significantly higher than the level of 1.3 ± 0.37 ng/ml of the control group ($p < 0.001$).

Similarly, the glycoside level in myocardium of patients with arrhythmias (97 ± 25.5 ng/g) was significantly higher than that of patients without arrhythmia (60 ± 15.2 ng/g). It should be noted that a ratio between tissue and serum glycoside levels was 50 : 1 in these studies, with no difference between the toxic and non-toxic groups of patients. This finding indirectly suggests that there is a linear relationship between serum glycoside level and the binding of the glycoside to its receptor in both the therapeutic and toxic range.

The relationship between serum glycoside levels and various effects is true not only for the therapeutic but also for the toxic range. Shown in Table 1, the danger of arrhythmias increases with increasing serum glycoside levels. 246 patients with rhythm disturbances during digoxin therapy were studied. 44 patients with ventricular extrasystole had an average serum glycoside level of 2.9 ± 0.59 ng/ml, 17 patients with a dangerous atrial tachycardia with block had an average level of 4.4 ± 2.04 ng/ml, 9 patients with third degree A-V block had a level of 5.4 ± 2.15 ng/ml, and 7 patients with ventricular fibrillation had an average level of 6.3 ± 3.55 ng/ml (11).

*Prof. A. Bohle, Pathological Institute of the University of Tübingen and Prof. H. E. Hoffmeister, Department of Cardiovascular Surgery at the University of Tübingen, are thanked for kindly supplying the tissue samples.

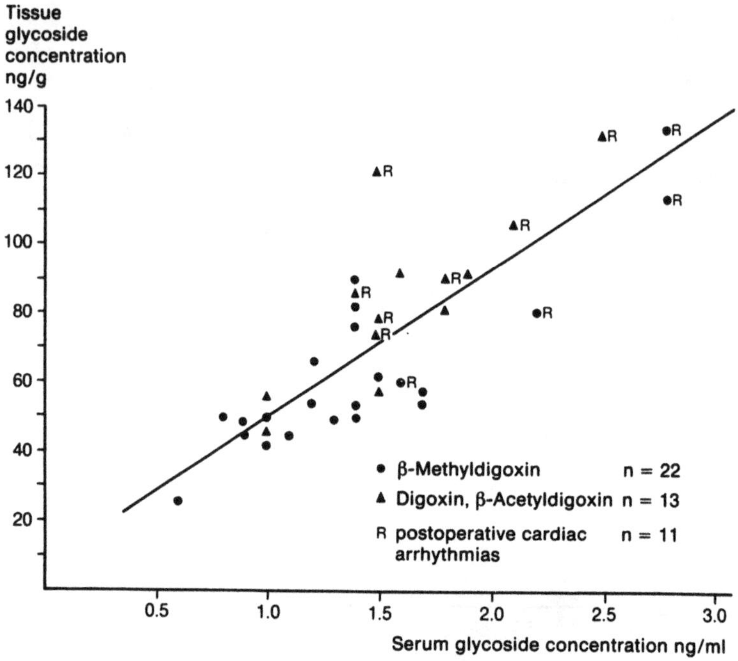

Fig. 2. Correlation between glycoside concentration in left ventricular papillary muscle and serum in 35 patients during cardiac surgery (prosthetic mitral valve replacement); $r = 0.814$; $p < 0.001$ (17).

Although studies on large numbers of patients have shown that there is a clear relationship between serum glycoside level and the severity of rhythm disorders, countless studies have demonstrated that this relationship cannot be established in an individual case. We examined the serum glycoside level in 1674 patients with no signs of glycoside intoxication and in 344 patients with signs of glycoside intoxication. All patients received digitalis maintenance therapy, suggesting a steady state condition. Serum glycoside levels were between 0.3–3.8 ng/ml (with a maximum of 1.0–1.3 ng/ml) in the non-toxic group, whereas the levels were 0.6–10.0 ng/ml (with a maximum of 3.8 ng/ml) in the toxic group. It was not possible to clearly distinguish the two groups using serum glycoside levels (17).

The region of overlap was between 0.6–3.8 ng/ml (fig. 3). However, the occurrence of toxicity with glycoside concentrations below 2.0 ng/ml was relatively infrequent whereas it increases steeply above this level. With a level of 3.8 ng/ml every patient displayed signs of toxicity. The cause of toxicity due to digoxin and its derivatives was decreased renal function in almost 70% of patients, 60% of the patients were older than 65 years of age, 16% had reduced body weight, and only 13% had received a true overdose therapy (17). These factors alone cannot explain the relatively broad region of overlap of the serum glycoside levels of the toxic and non-toxic groups. For some time, it has been known that the digitalis sensitivity of patients can differ, for which there are few pharmacological explanations. Hypercalcemia (19), hypokalemia (18) and hypomagnesemia (20) diminish, hypocalcemia (5), hyperkalemia (8), and hypermagnesemia (3) increase the digitalis tolerance. Responsiveness to digitalis is diminished by the hyperthyroid state and increased by the hypothyroid state (6). Both, acidosis (10) and alkalosis (21) are suggested to decrease digitalis tolerance.

Table 1. Toxic cardiac arrhythmias and serum glycoside concentrations in 246 cases of glycoside intoxication with digoxin and digoxin derivatives confirmed by electrocardiography (17).

Type of arrhythmia	Number	%	Serum glycoside concentration ng/ml (x ± SD)
AV block I	61	25	3.2 ± 0.86
Ventricular extrasystoles	44	18	2.9 ± 0.59
Atrial fibrillation with bradycardia (Ventricular rate <55/min)	28	11	3.5 ± 1.58
Ventricular bigeminy	25	10	3.4 ± 1.40
AV block II	17	7	3.9 ± 1.68
Type I (Wenckebach)	12		4.1 ± 1.91
Type II (Mobitz)	5		3.4 ± 1.15
Atrial tachycardia with block (PAT)	17	7	4.4 ± 2.04
AV block III	9	4	5.4 ± 2.15
Sinus bradycardia	8	3	2.8 ± 0.50
Nodal rhythm	7	3	3.7 ± 1.21
Supraventricular extrasystoles	7	3	3.1 ± 0.87
Ventricular fibrillation	7	3	6.3 ± 3.35
Sinoatrial block	6	2	4.3 ± 1.33
Ventricular tachycardia	4	2	4.0 ± 1.06
AV dissociation	3	1	4.2 ± 1.29
Left-bundle branch block	2	1	2.8 ± 0.21
Supraventricular tachycardia	1	0.5	3.3

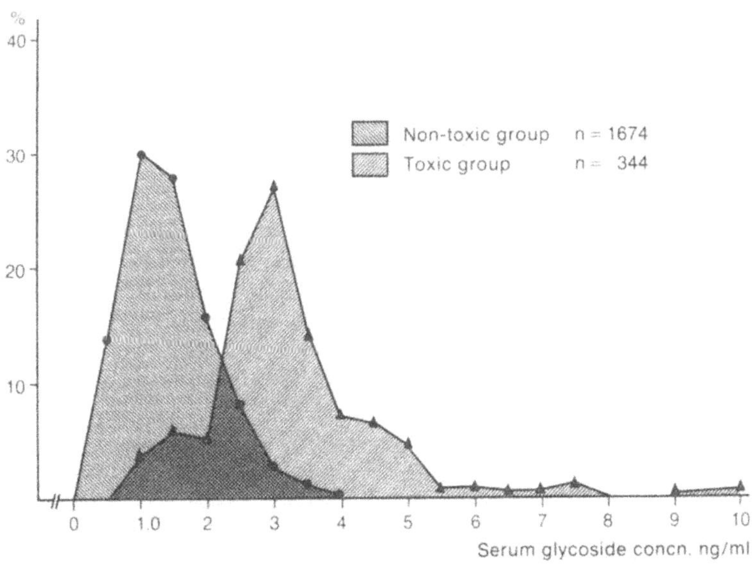

Fig. 3. Percentage distribution of serum glycoside concentrations in 1674 patients without toxic symptoms and 344 patients with symptoms of intoxication. Overlapping range: 0.6–3.8 ng/ml (17).

Of specific clinical relevance is the reduction of digitalis tolerance by hypoxia and hypoxemia. Of our 246 patients with digitalis intoxication, 31, or 12%, died of their digitalis intoxication, including 9 who suffered from cor pulmonale. At the time of death, these 9 patients had glycoside levels of 3.3 ng/ml which was significantly lower than the level of 5.1 ng/ml measured in the other 22 patients who died (17). A diminished digitalis tolerance can also be found in patients with coronary heart disease, and in addition it has long been known that severely diseased hearts are especially sensitive to digitalis (2). It has been suspected, although not clearly demonstrated, that regional differences in myocardial hypoxia and acidosis with subsequent loss of cellular potassium is responsible for this phenomenon (9). Also increased sympathetic activity is accompanied by diminished digitalis tolerance (22). Unexplained at present is the relative digitalis insensitivity in atrial fibrillation. Patients with atrial fibrillation tolerate much higher serum glycoside levels and develop immediately glycoside toxicity when a sinus rhythm returns (7, 15).

At the beginning of the paper the difficulties in defining the therapeutic range in the clinical setting was discussed. In the clinic, only the upper limit of the therapeutic range (for example, when undesired side effects begin) can be recognized with some degree of certainty. Therefore, if relatively high serum glycoside levels are tolerated without side effects (for example, above 2.0 ng/ml digoxin or above 30 ng/ml digitoxin), this can be considered an increased therapeutic range. The opposite applies to a decreased tolerance of serum glycoside levels. Since a decreased therapeutic range is very important clinically, because of the danger of intoxication, many studies have addressed this topic. Further examinations of patients who tolerate a relatively high serum glycoside level demonstrated that this was not the result of increased therapeutic range. In these patients, positive inotropic effects could also only be observed at relatively high glycoside levels (13). Such a shift of the therapeutic effect to a range of relatively high serum glycoside levels has been demonstrated to occur with both hypocalcemia and hyperkalemia, and has been demonstrated as a result of the stabilizing effects of diphenylhydantoin (14) and possibly β-receptor blockers.

Summarized from the standpoint of a clinician, there is no evidence that the small therapeutic range can be increased for the effective cardiac glycosides which act by inhibiting the sodium-potassium ATPase. Although certain drugs, hormones, and changes in electrolytes (such as potassium, calcium and magnesium) may shift the therapeutic range of glycosides to high serum glycoside levels, an increase in the therapeutic range is not achieved in such situations. A true increase in therapeutic range may be present in absolute tachyarrhythmia and in a hyperthyroid state. Also, in childhood (after the first month of life) digitalis tolerance appears to be increased, the cause of which is unknown.

In the clinic, glycosides with a short elimination half-life are said to have an increased therapeutic range. Practically, this appears to be true no doubt because toxic symptoms disappear sooner. However, at the time of maximal effect, the therapeutic range does not appear to differ from other glycosides. A practical disadvantage of glycosides with a short elimination half-life is the necessity of using several daily doses. Furthermore, these glycosides are eliminated by the kidney, such that impaired renal function will have important pharmacokinetic consequences.

Meproscillarin, which has a short elimination half-life independent of renal function, may be an alternative, although this cannot be decided at present due to insufficient pharmacological and clinical evidence (4).

The question raised by the topic of this paper can be answered from the standpoint of a clinician as follows: The therapeutic range of effective cardiac glycosides is determined by their pharmacodynamic and pharmacokinetic properties. The pharmacodynamic properties appear to be identical for all known glycosides, whereas the glycosides can be distinguished by their pharmacokinetic properties. Countless endogenous and exogenous factors are able to modify the pharmacodynamic and pharmacokinetic parameters. A true increase in therapeutic range, however, cannot be reached.

Finally, I wish to acknowledge that the studies of our own group have been carried out by my former colleagues Dr. Larbig and Dr. Haasis.

References

1. Bahrmann H, Greeff K (1981) Evaluation of cardiac glycosides in the intact animal. In: Greef K (ed): Cardiac glycosides. Part I (Springer Verlag, Berlin–Heidelberg–New York) p 138
2. Beller GA, Smith TW, Abelman WH, Haber E, Hood WB (1971) Digitalis intoxication. A prospective clinical study with serum level correlations. New Engl J Med 284:989
3. Beller GA, Hood WB, Senita TW, Abelman WH, Wacker WEC (1974) Correlation of serum magnesium levels and cardiac digitalis intoxication. Am J Cardiol 33:225
4. Belz GG, Schreiber H, Wolf KG (1976) Pharmacokinetics and pharmacodynamics of methylproscillaridin in healthy man. Eur J Clin Pharmacol 10:101
5. Chopra D, Janson P, Sawin CT (1977) Insensitivity to digoxin with hypocalcaemia. New Engl J Med 296:917
6. Doherty JE, Perkins WH (1966) Digoxin metablism in hypo- and hyperthyreoidism. Ann Intern Med 64:489
7. Elkins RC, Vasko JS, Marrow AG (1967) Digitalis: tolerance during atrial fibrillation and normal sinus rhythm. Am J Cardiol 20:229
8. Goldman RH, Coltart DJ, Friedman JP, Gaeton TN, Berke DK, Schweizer E, Harrison DC (1973) The inotropic effects of digoxin in hyperkalemia. Relation to (Na^+,K^+)-ATPase. Inhibition in the intact animal. Circulation 48:830
9. Goldsmith C, Kapadia GG, Numino L (1969) Correlation of digitalis intoxication with myocardial concentration of triated digoxin in hypokalemia and normokalemic dog (Abstr.) Circulation 40:III–92
10. Green LH, Smith TW (1977) The use of digitalis in patients with pulmonary disease. Ann Intern Med 87:459
11. Haasis R, Larbig D (1975) Serumglykosidkonzentration und Digitalisintoxikation. Dtsch med Wschr 100:1768
12. Haasis R, Larbig D, Schubert R, Becker H, Seboldt H (1977) Radioimmunologische Bestimmung der Glykosidkonzentration in menschlichem Gewebe. Klin Wschr 55:23
13. Hayes CJ, Butler VP jr, Gersony WM (1973) Serum digoxin studies in infants and children. Pediat 52:561
14. Helfant RH, Scherlag BJ, Damato AN (1967) The electrophysiological properties of diphenylhydantoin sodium as compared to procaine amid in the normal and digitalis-intoxicated heart. Circulation 36:108
15. Larbig D, Kochsiek K, Schrader Chr (1972) Klinische Aspekte der radioimmunchemischen Bestimmung der Serum-Digoxin Konzentration. Dtsch med Wschr 97:139
16. Larbig D, Haasis R (1975) Radioimmunologische Bestimmung der Konzentration von Digoxin und Digoxinderivaten. In: Digitalistherapie (Hrsg. Jahrmärker, H) Springer Verlag, Berlin–Heidelberg–New York p 62
17. Larbig D, Haasis R, Kochsiek K (1978) The glycoside concentration and its clinical significance. Forum cardiologicum 15, Boehringer Mannheim, p 76
18. Mason DT, Zelis R, Lee G (1971) Current concepts and treatment of digitalis toxicity. Am J Cardiol 27:546
19. Nola GT, Pope S, Harrison DC (1970) Assessment of the synergistic relationship between serum calcium and digitalis. Am Heart J 79:499
20. Seller RH, Cangiano J, Kim KE (1970) Digitalis toxicity and hypermagnesemia. Am Heart J 79:57
21. Warren MC, Cianelly RE, Cutler SL, Harrison DC (1968) Digitalis toxicity, II. The effect of metabolic alkalosis. Am Heart J 75:358

22. Weaver LC, Akera T, Broody TM (1976) Digoxin toxicity, Primary site of drug action on the sympathetic nervous system. J Pharmacol Exp Ther 197:1

Author's address:

Prof. Dr. K. Kochsiek, Med. Univ. Klinik, Luitpoldkrankenhaus, Josef-Schneider-Straße 2, D 8700 Würzburg (FRG)

Authors' Index

Subject Index

www.ingramcontent.com/pod-product-compliance
Lightning Source LLC
Chambersburg PA
CBHW061215240926
51846CB00006B/1232
* 9 7 8 3 6 4 2 7 2 3 7 8 0 *